Keto Friendly Recipes

~~~

BAKE IT

KETO

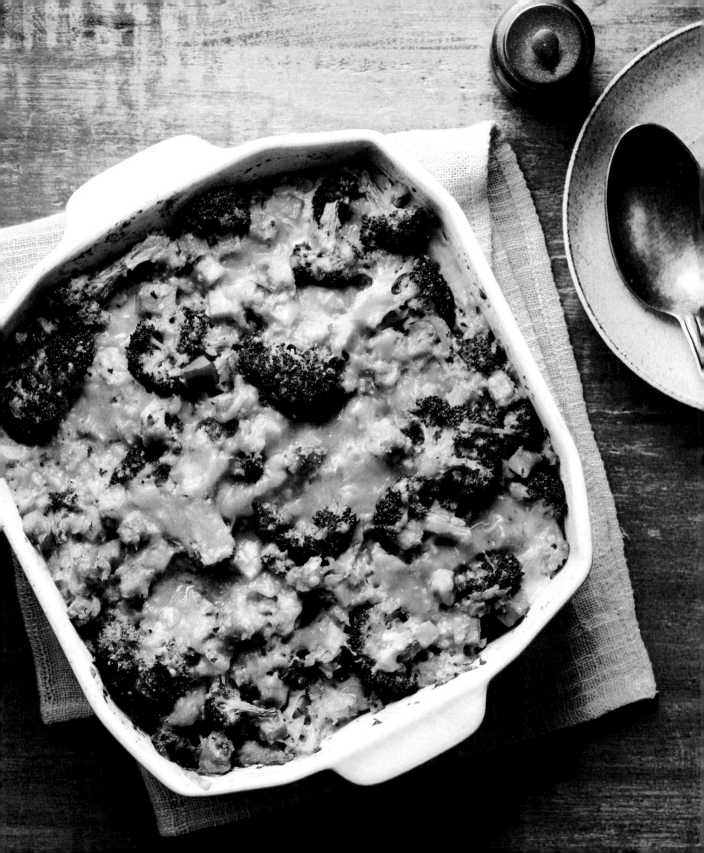

Keto Friendly
Recipes

~~~

BAKE IT
KETO

~~~

JENNIFER MARIE GARZA
of Keto Friendly Recipes and Low Carb Inspirations

Photography by Ghazalle Badiozamani

HOUGHTON MIFFLIN HARCOURT
BOSTON NEW YORK 2020

For information about permission to reproduce selections from this book, write
to trade.permissions@hmhco.com or to Permissions, Houghton Mifflin Harcourt
Publishing Company, 3 Park Avenue, 19th Floor, New York, New York 10016.
hmhbooks.com

Library of Congress Cataloging-in-Publication Data
Names: Garza, Jennifer Marie, author.
Title: Keto friendly recipes : bake it keto / Jennifer Marie Garza.
Description: Boston : Houghton Mifflin Harcourt, 2020. | Includes index. |
    Summary: "Sweet and savory keto breads, cakes, muffins, bagels, cookies,
    pizza, doughnuts, and more from the best-selling author of Keto Friendly
    Recipes: Easy Keto for Busy People"-- Provided by publisher.
Identifiers: LCCN 2020003645 (print) | LCCN 2020003646 (ebook) |
    ISBN 9780358346883 (trade paperback) | ISBN 9780358350798 (ebook)
Subjects: LCSH: Low-carbohydrate diet--Recipes. | Baking. |
    LCGFT: Cookbooks.
Classification: LCC RM237.73 .G373 2020 (print) | LCC RM237.73 (ebook) |
    DDC 641.5/6383--dc23
LC record available at https://lccn.loc.gov/2020003645
LC ebook record available at https://lccn.loc.gov/2020003646

Book design by Allison Chi
Printed in the United States of America
DOC 10 9 8 7 6 5 4 3 2 1

To my fans who love food just as much as I do.
To my husband, John, who is always willing to help me even when
he works a stressful, full-time job of his own. I love you!
To my daughters, Megan and Melanie, who are not afraid to give me
their honest opinions about anything I ask them to test.

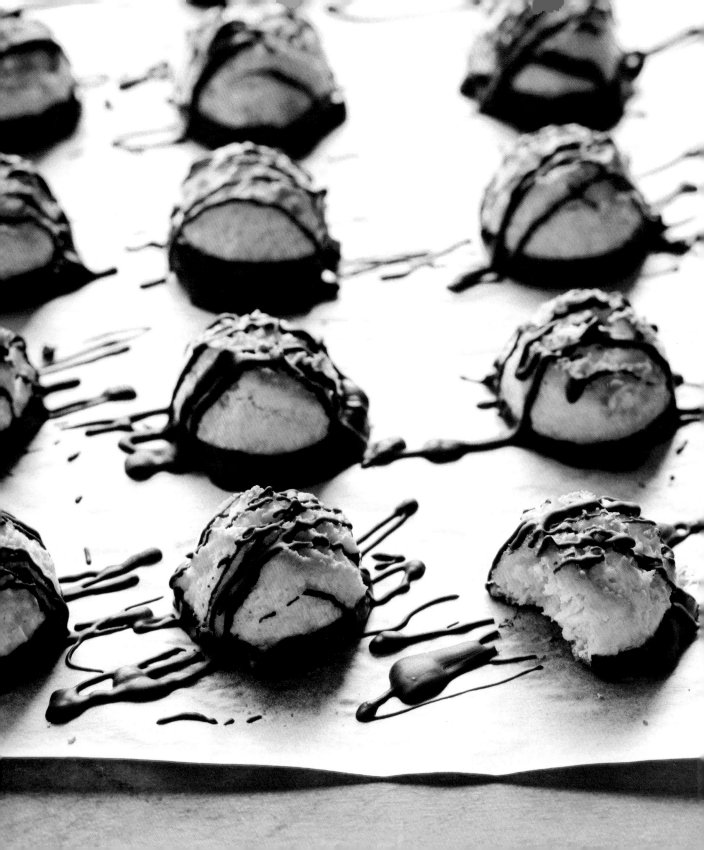

CONTENTS

〜〜〜〜

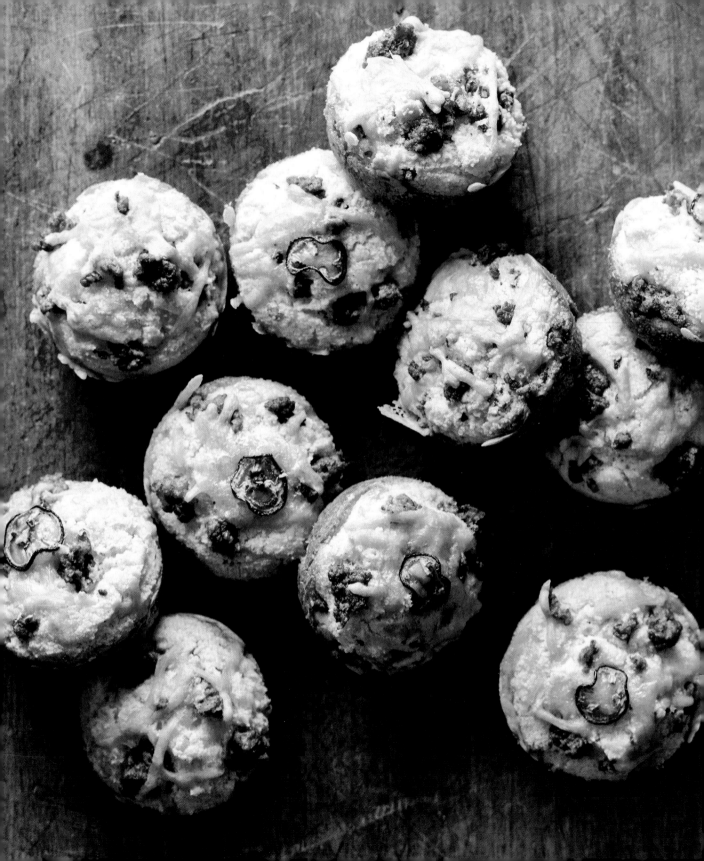

Acknowledgments

To my editor, Justin Schwartz, thank you for believing in me. It is always a pleasure to work with you and I'm blessed to work with the best in the business!

To my agent, Lisa Grubka, thank you for helping me understand this process and giving me your valuable advice.

To my editor, Amy Treadwell, a huge thank you for helping me express exactly what I was trying to say. I could not have done this without you. You have a true talent!

Special thanks to Ghazalle Badiozamani for the photography, Barrett Washburne for the food styling, and Jenna Tedesco for the prop styling.

To my family: my husband, John, and my beautiful daughters, Megan and Melanie, I am so thankful that you have supported me on this journey to create another cookbook. I could not have done this without all of your ideas, recipe testing, and the chores you took over to take some of the work off my hands. Thank you for always supporting me in everything I do!

To Mom, Dad, and brother Raymond, thank you for your love and support.

To Andrea Deckard, thank you for always being there for me. I am forever grateful for your friendship and guidance.

To Kristi Reddell, thank you for being my sidekick in everything I do. You are such a hard worker and I am very grateful to have you on my team.

To Vanessa Minton, thank you for all your help in the kitchen. I am grateful for the knowledge you have given me. You are a beautiful and talented person.

To the members of the Low Carb Inspirations group and Keto Chaffle Recipes group on Facebook, thank you for being part of an online community that has helped me through my own journey. I hope to return the positivity tenfold. Special thanks to Becky Grimmer, Michelle Ierna, Cheryl Williams, Shari Williams, Tammi Lemons, Christy Wilkins Rowell, Diana Wilson Peters, Bryan Foulk, and Kris Dee for helping to moderate such an uplifting group of low-carb and keto people. You are always willing to help other people on their journey and I'm happy to know you. You guys are the best!

To the members of the Beef and Butter Fast 5-Day Challenge Facebook Group, thank you for trusting me and my crazy process to help you get out of a keto weight loss stall.

And last, but not least, thank you to everyone who follows my Low Carb Inspirations blog. Your comments and questions keep my desire going! I am forever grateful.

Introduction

〜〜〜〜〜〜

Welcome! My name is Jennifer Marie and I've been on the ketogenic diet for three years now. I've lost 55 pounds and I've kept it off. I started eating this way to lose weight, but after learning about all the other benefits of a keto diet, it quickly became a way of life for me and my family.

I remember vividly what it was like at the beginning of my journey. The food seemed foreign to me and I questioned my self-determination. I remember saying out loud, "How long will I stick to this diet?" I know what it's like to try multiple diets in an effort to lose weight, only to fail every time. I didn't think I had the willpower that others seemed to have. I questioned, "Why am I so weak in this process?"

I wish I could go back and have someone reassure me that this process would change my life!

I wish someone had told me that it was never about willpower!

I wish someone had told me how brave I was to start this new way of life!

I wish someone had told me that even though I failed at so many other diets, the ketogenic diet would be the one I would stick to.

But now I know. This is no longer just a diet for me. This is my way of life. The ketogenic way of eating has changed my life and it will change yours too. Let me be the person who tells you that it's not about willpower. You are brave and you can succeed, even if you don't believe that in the beginning.

I created the site LowCarbInspirations.com to share my recipes with whoever wanted them. I never imagined that I would be helping millions of people each month!

Many people have reached out to me and even sent letters about how the keto diet and my first cookbook, *Keto Friendly Recipes: Easy Keto for Busy People,* has helped them. It seems as though every day I get new messages from readers telling me that their life has been changed.

I truly enjoy creating delicious keto-friendly meals and treats for my friends and family. It has been my calling to help those of you on this journey, and this cookbook is meant to continue the work my website and book have already been doing—guiding those traveling on the road to ketosis. I hope you will enjoy these recipes as much as I do.

ABOUT THE KETO DIET

The ketogenic diet is a way of eating that allows your body to burn ketones as its main fuel source. Your body can burn either glucose or ketones. If you are eating foods from the Standard American Diet (SAD), you are probably burning glucose, or are what we might call a "sugar burner."

By simply limiting your carbohydrate and sugar intake, you can switch your body's fuel source from glucose to ketones; that's when you start to lose weight. Some people can burn ketones while consuming 100 grams of carbs a day, while others may have to be way stricter and limit their carb intake to about 20 grams of carbs per day. The difference depends on your metabolic health. I suffer from insulin resistance so my carb intake must be 20 grams or lower to be sure that I stay in a ketogenic state.

The keto diet is an excellent choice for those who need to lose weight, but there are other reasons to go keto. The keto diet has helped people with everything from reducing chronic pain and inflammation, lowering A1C or blood pressure, and even slowing the effects in those suffering from brain diseases such as Alzheimer's and dementia.

The very first thing I tell people when they want to start keto is to start slow and do what they are comfortable with in the beginning. The average American eating the SAD diet consumes an average of 200 to 250 grams of carbs a day.

If you start by reducing your carbohydrate intake and cutting out the sugar, that would already be a huge improvement from what you are probably used to eating.

I always tell people that I was the most sugar-addicted person on the planet. No one loved sugar more than I did. I haven't had sugar in three years and I no longer feel controlled by sugar or controlled by food in general. It's a great feeling. I don't consider the keto diet to be a fad. There are way too many benefits to this way of eating for it to go away any time soon.

Once you start talking with people about the keto diet, you will find that there are many different versions of this way of eating. Some people will be completely strict and eat a very clean keto diet by keeping their macros under 20 carbs a day and eating only whole foods. Others may follow a more relaxed keto regimen by not worrying so much about sugar alcohols or the types of foods they are eating as long as they fit in within their macronutrient goals.

My husband, John, is in the relaxed category. He cannot give up his diet soda, which does not belong on a strict keto diet, so he follows what would be considered a more relaxed keto diet, or "lazy keto" as it is sometimes called. He doesn't battle the insulin resistance issues I do, though he continues to have lower inflammation, and he has lost 80 pounds to date!

I run a large Facebook group called Low Carb Inspirations (plus Keto Friendly Recipes) facebook.com/groups/lowcarbinspirations. In these types of social groups you will hear the keto diet referred to by many different terms depending on how strict or lenient you are with your food choices. They all work for different individuals and you will need to choose what works best for you.

Keto Plans

STRICT KETO: This is someone who is very strict with their food choices and keeps their carb intake to 20 grams or less per day. This person will probably use a meal tracking app to help them keep on target. It's a great plan for those who love to track their progress.

LAZY KETO: This person will count carbohydrates and stay under 20 grams per day, but they won't use a meal tracking device and they won't count calories. They will focus solely on the limit of carbs. This method is best for people who prefer simplicity and hate tracking.

DIRTY KETO: This person will only count carbohydrates and stay under 20 grams of carbs or less per day. This person is less focused on whole foods and may consider eating processed foods or slightly more unhealthy choices as long as that keeps them within their goals. This is perfect for someone who finds eating clean difficult, but still wants to achieve their weight loss goal.

Here's the thing: There are many ways to follow the keto diet and it's up to you to find the way that works best for you. I found that the hardest part of the diet was finding delicious meals I enjoyed eating, and that is why I created this cookbook.

Once you start eating keto and you become more comfortable with your food choices, you will notice that you will naturally be less hungry. Being less hungry will allow you to stay true to your goals.

I've helped many people transition to the keto way of life. I almost always see the same thing. Most people want to make a keto version of their favorite pre-diet foods. It helps them feel as though they aren't missing out on anything.

Then, their palate starts to change and foods start to taste different. They notice that berries are all of a sudden really sweet. They begin to enjoy the flavors of the seasonings too. They notice that they are eating less and don't require the same amount of food they did when they weren't limiting carbs and sugar intake. They start to get really excited about the weight loss or the lowered inflammation that lessens their pain, and start to become more strict as they continue on their keto journey.

That is why there are so many versions of this diet that actually work. It depends on where you are on your own journey and what goals you want to accomplish.

You will no longer think about sugar and bread because you'll discover the many wonderful low-carb and keto bread options available.

Keto Flu

The keto diet is considered a flushing diet because when you begin, it immediately reduces inflammation, which causes water

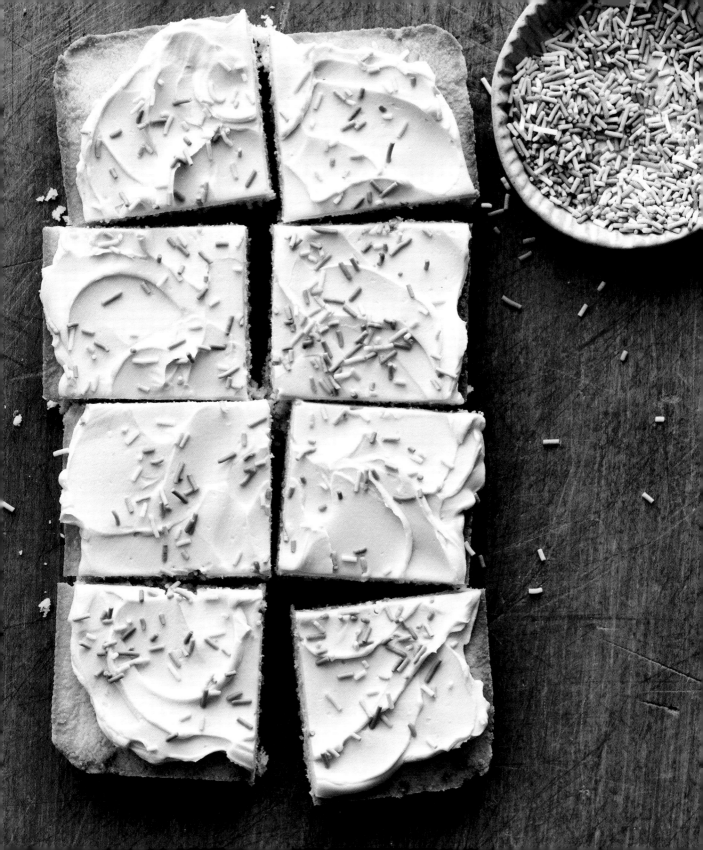

to release. When you lose a lot of water, you also lose minerals. That is why supplementing with electrolytes in the beginning is extremely important.

If you have an electrolyte imbalance you might feel dizzy, nauseated, lightheaded, or even have a racing heartbeat. These are all clear signs of keto flu and that you need to supplement with electrolytes.

The keto flu is avoidable! In addition to taking an electrolyte supplement, you should consume extra pink Himalayan salt. And you'll need additional calcium, magnesium, potassium, and sodium. I suggest pink salt because it contains about 84 different minerals that the body needs. The salt will also help to hold in some of the liquids that you lose in the beginning. Even after following this diet for three years, I still consume extra pink salt for the beneficial minerals.

How to Know If You're Fat Adapted

When you no longer think about food, that's a good sign that you are fat adapted. You might be able to skip a normal scheduled meal. You might eat breakfast and realize you are not even hungry for lunch. You will have much more energy too. I felt like I could run all around my neighborhood and I had not run in years!

How to Prep Ahead of Time When You Are Busy

I've discovered a few tips that will help get dinner on the table quickly and without fuss.

- There are lots of casseroles in this book that are super-easy to put together.
- Cook all the meats you planned for the week on Sunday and turn them into different meals during the week.
- Keep your freezer stocked with frozen microwavable vegetables.
- Rediscover your waffle maker. There are several recipes for savory and sweet chaffles that will take only a few minutes to make.

To Track or Not to Track Macros

I always suggest that people track their foods at the beginning of their journey. It's shocking how much sugar is hidden in the foods we consume every day. Once you are really comfortable with your food choices, I don't see the need to track it closely. Success happens when you become comfortable in choosing what you eat and it becomes second nature.

Don't forget: Hidden sugars are everywhere. Question everything. Always read the labels.

Keto Is a State Your Body Is In, It Is Not a Food

Remember, ketosis is a state in which your body is burning ketones. Keto is not a food. The number of carbs and sugar you should eat will depend on whether or not your body is in a state of ketosis.

Different people can eat different macro-nutrients counts and still maintain ketosis. For example, kids, who are naturally more active, can easily eat 100 grams of carbs and still be in ketosis. There are foods that are considered keto friendly because of the types of keto friendly sweeteners used or the quality of carbohydrates—such as those you find in healthy vegetables. The amount of those foods you should eat for your body to be in ketosis will depend on your own metabolism. You will easily figure this out by testing your glucose and ketone readings with a blood glucose/ketone meter.

BAKING ON THE KETO DIET

There are a few ingredients I use frequently when baking keto recipes:

UNFLAVORED COLLAGEN PEPTIDES. Collagen is an excellent source of protein and contains several essential amino acids. Collagen peptides are broken down a bit more than regular collagen, which helps aid digestion. These peptides do not gel when mixed with liquid like regular collagen does; instead they dissolve, which works well in baking. Collagen peptides help curb sugar cravings but that's not the only reason I'm a big fan. They also improve digestion, reduce inflammation, and hydrate your skin. They are safe to cook and bake with, and I have found that adding some creates a moist texture in many of my baked goods.

OAT FIBER. This is not the same as oat flour, so I don't want you to get the two confused. Oat fiber is the outside layer of the oat grain. It consists mainly of lignin, cellulose, and hemicellulose, which is a rich source of insoluble dietary fiber. This fiber is gluten free and non-digestible. It has a very fine texture and it makes most of my baked goods taste like real bread or real cake! It's definitely an ingredient I've added to my keto pantry.

PSYLLIUM HUSK. Use this fiber ground or whole. The whole husk is nondigestible and the ground husk is only partially digestible. The psyllium husk helps to retain moisture and keeps baked goods from being too crumbly.

FLAXSEED. This is a rich source of healthy fat, antioxidants, and fiber, and it's gluten free. Whole flaxseed is nondigestible while ground flaxseed is only partially digestible. It is coarse in texture and makes an excellent binder in recipes, and it can replace eggs in some recipes.

CHIA SEEDS. Loaded with important nutrients and an excellent source of omega-3 fatty acids, chia is rich in antioxidants, fiber, iron, and calcium. Chia seeds can be used as an egg replacement in some recipes. They work as a binder in baked goods and can be a thickener for sauces.

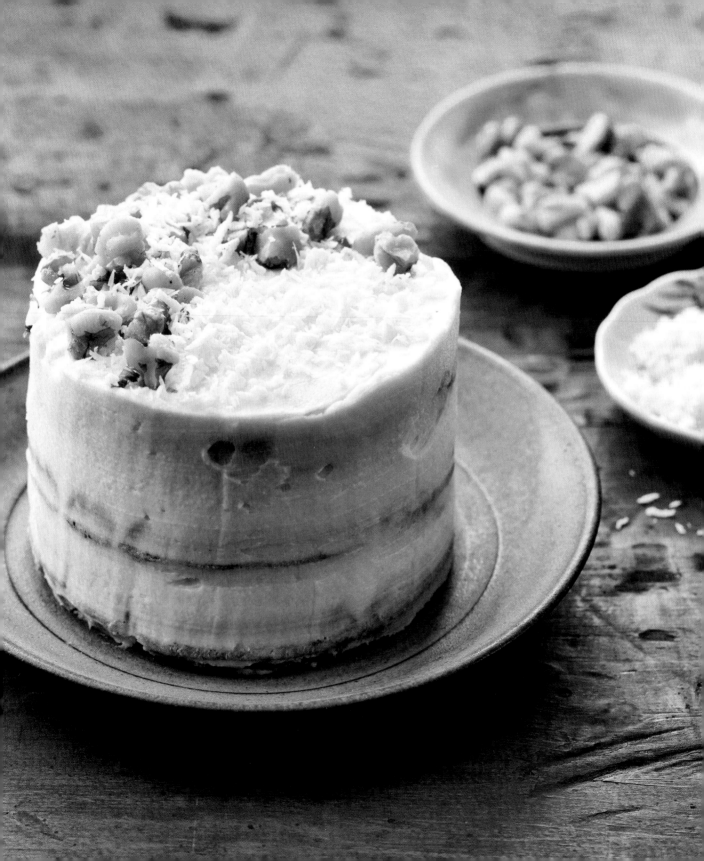

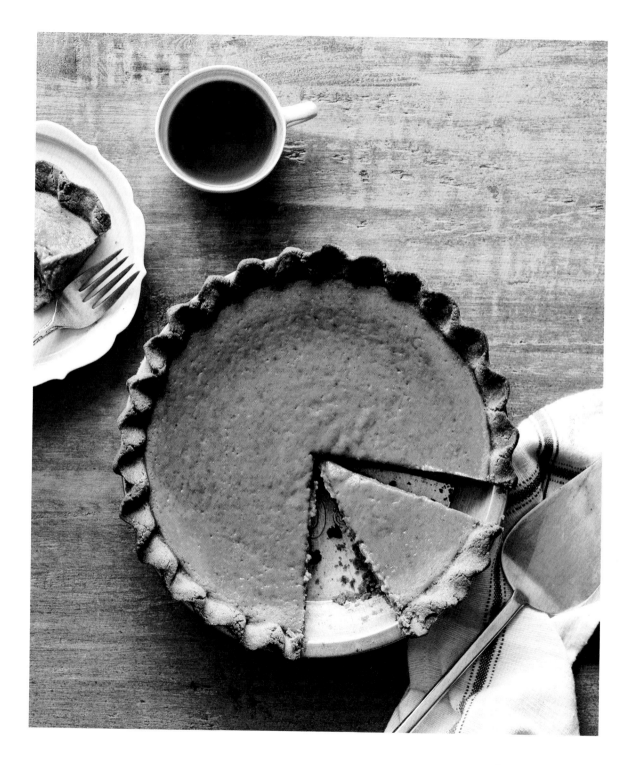

KETO BAKING GUIDE

Use the following charts as a reference to help you choose the right ingredients, depending on the recipe you are making. Keto baking can be difficult, especially when you have to substitute an ingredient. This guide was designed to help you understand the ingredients and how they work when you bake with them.

FIBER

	GLUTEN FREE	DIGESTIBLE	EGG REPLACEMENT	PREBIOTIC	TEXTURE
OAT FIBER	Yes	No	No	No	Fine
PSYLLIUM HUSK, WHOLE	Yes	No	No	No	Coarse
PSYLLIUM HUSK, GROUND	Yes	Partially digestible	No	No	Coarse
YACON ROOT	Yes	No	No	Yes	Syrup
FLAXSEED, WHOLE	Yes	No	Yes	Yes	Coarse
FLAXSEED, GROUND	Yes	Partially digestible	Yes	Yes	Coarse
CHICORY ROOT	Yes	No	No	No	Fine
INULIN	Yes	No	No	Yes	Fine
KONJAC (GLUCOMANNAN)	Yes	No	No	No	Fine
CHIA SEEDS	Yes	No	Yes	Yes	Coarse

STABILIZERS

	ADDS MOISTURE	ADDS PROTEIN	ADDS CRUNCHY TEXTURE	ADDS CHEWY TEXTURE	GLUTEN FREE
VITAL WHEAT GLUTEN	n/a	Yes	No	Yes	No
COLLAGEN PEPTIDES	Yes	Yes	No	No	Yes
COLLAGEN	Yes	Yes	No	No	Yes
WHEY PROTEIN ISOLATE	No	Yes	Yes	No	Yes
XANTHAN GUM	n/a	No	Yes	Yes	Yes
GUAR GUM	n/a	No	No	Yes	Yes
GELATIN	Yes	Yes	No	No	Yes

FLOUR NUTRITIONAL VALUES

PER ¼ CUP	CARBS	FIBER	NET CARBS	PROTEIN	CALORIES	FAT
BLANCHED ALMOND FLOUR	12g	6g	6g	12g	320	28g
COCONUT FLOUR	16g	10g	6g	4g	120	4g
LUPIN FLOUR	24g	22g	2g	24g	148	4g
PECAN FLOUR	3g	1g	1g	1g	133	15g
WALNUT FLOUR	3g	1g	1g	3g	130	13g
RAW PUMPKIN SEED FLOUR	5g	3g	2g	10g	130	17.4g
SUNFLOWER SEED FLOUR	5g	0.8g	4.2g	7g	52	0.3g

FLOUR BAKING QUALITIES

	TASTE	LIGHT OR HEAVY IN RECIPES	TEXTURE	ABSORBS LIQUIDS	NUT FREE	
BLANCHED ALMOND FLOUR	Nutty	Heavy	Coarse	No	No	
COCONUT FLOUR	Mild coconut flavor	Light	Coarse	Yes	Yes	
LUPIN FLOUR	Bitter	Light	Fine	Yes	Yes	
PECAN FLOUR	Nutty	Heavy	Coarse	No	No	
WALNUT FLOUR	Nutty	Heavy	Coarse	No	No	
RAW PUMPKIN SEED FLOUR	Earthy	Heavy	Less coarse	No	Yes	
SUNFLOWER SEED FLOUR	Earthy	Heavy	Less coarse	No	Yes	
PORK RINDS	Savory	Heavy	Crunchy	Yes	Yes	
TAPIOCA STARCH	Neutral	Light	Fine	Yes	Yes	

	BEST TO USE WITH OTHER FLOURS	USE STAND-ALONE WITH NO OTHER FLOURS	USE AS A BREADING	USE IN BAKED GOODS	USE AS A THICKENER	BROWNS EASILY
	n/a	Yes	Yes	Yes	Yes	Yes
	Yes	Yes	No	Yes	Yes	Yes
	Yes	No	No	Yes	Yes	No
	n/a	Yes	Yes	Yes	Yes	Yes
	n/a	Yes	Yes	Yes	Yes	Yes
	n/a	Yes	n/a	Yes	Yes	No
	n/a	Yes	n/a	Yes	Yes	No
	n/a	n/a	Yes	Yes	No	No
	Yes	No	No	Yes	Yes	No

KETO SWEETENERS

	PERCENTAGE OF SWEETNESS COMPARED TO SUGAR	CRYSTALLIZED	BROWNS	AFTERTASTE	BAKED GOOD TEXTURE	OK TO USE AS A STAND-ALONE SWEETENER IN RECIPE	
ERYTHRITOL	70%	Yes	No	Cooling	Firm and dry	Yes	
STEVIA	250%	No	No	Bitter	Seizes liquids	No, best in a blend	
MONKFRUIT	150%	Yes	No	Bitter	Seizes liquids	Yes	
XYLITOL	95%	No	No	Tangy	None	Yes	
ALLULOSE	70%	No	Yes	None	Makes baked goods soft and spreadable	Yes	
BOCHASWEET	100%	No	Yes	Small cooling	Makes baked goods soft and spreadable	Yes	
VEGETABLE GLYCERIN	40%	No	No	None	Prevents crystallization	No, best in a blend	

MAY CAUSE DIGESTIVE DISTRESS	TEXTURE	AVAILABLE AS GRANULAR	AVAILABLE AS POWDERED	AVAILABLE AS GOLDEN (BROWN)	AVAILABLE AS LIQUID	NOTE
Rarely	Medium granulation	Yes	Yes	Yes	No	Add mapleine extract to any sweetener to make it a golden-brown sugar blend.
No	Powdered fine	Yes	Yes	No	Yes	This sweetener is not to be used as a stand-alone sweetener and works better in a blend. Can make a sauce seize up. Liquid works best in drink recipes.
No	Powdered fine	Yes	Yes	Yes	Yes	Monkfruit concentrate is very bitter. It is often blended with erythritol. Doesn't have a cooling effect. Baking has little effect on the final texture. Pairing monkfruit with salt can balance out the sweetness. It can be used to round out the sweetness when paired with another sweetener.
No	Large granulation	Yes	No	No	No	Can have a tangy flavor in baked goods. Thick granulation that does not dissolve. Can be powdered in a food processor. Can make baked goods a little softer. Great for dusting or coating baked goods. Not good in liquids.
Yes	Fine granulation	Yes	No	No	Yes	Made from fermented corn. Closest thing to real sugar. Allows caramelization. Keeps recipes soft and pliable. Great for ice creams and sauces. Heated allulose can intensify gastric distress. Baking in small amounts is okay. Best combined with stevia and monkfruit to round out sweetness.
Yes (sometimes)	Small flake granulation	Yes	Yes	No	No	Comes from kabocha squash. Used in Asian cuisine. Keeps baked goods soft and pliable. Non-GMO. Can be used in a blend or on its own. It does caramelize but doesn't crystalize. Keeps baked goods softer but not as soft as allulose.
No	Liquid	No	No	No	Yes	Vegetable glycerin is a sugar alcohol derived from plants.

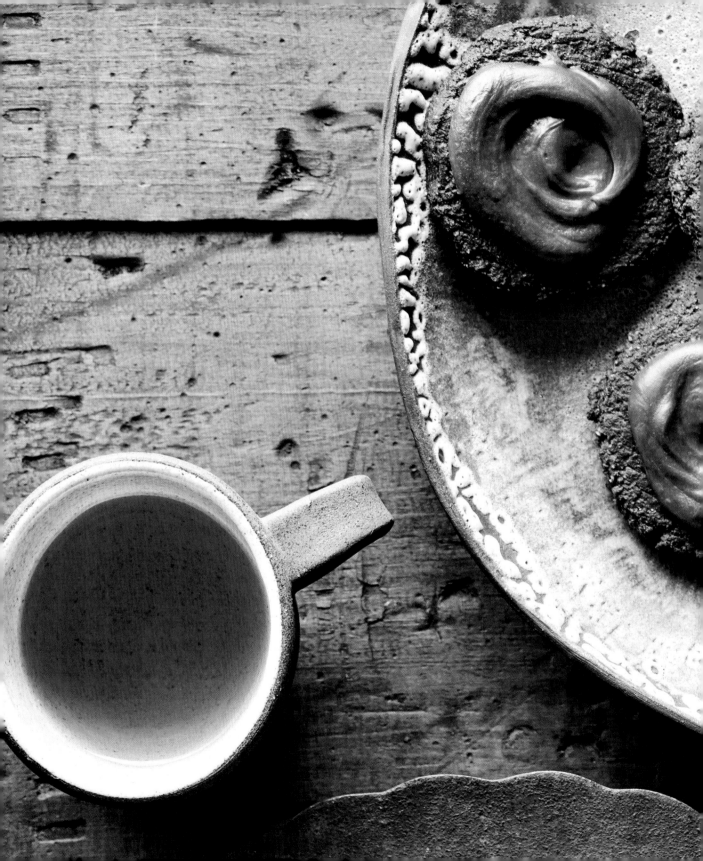

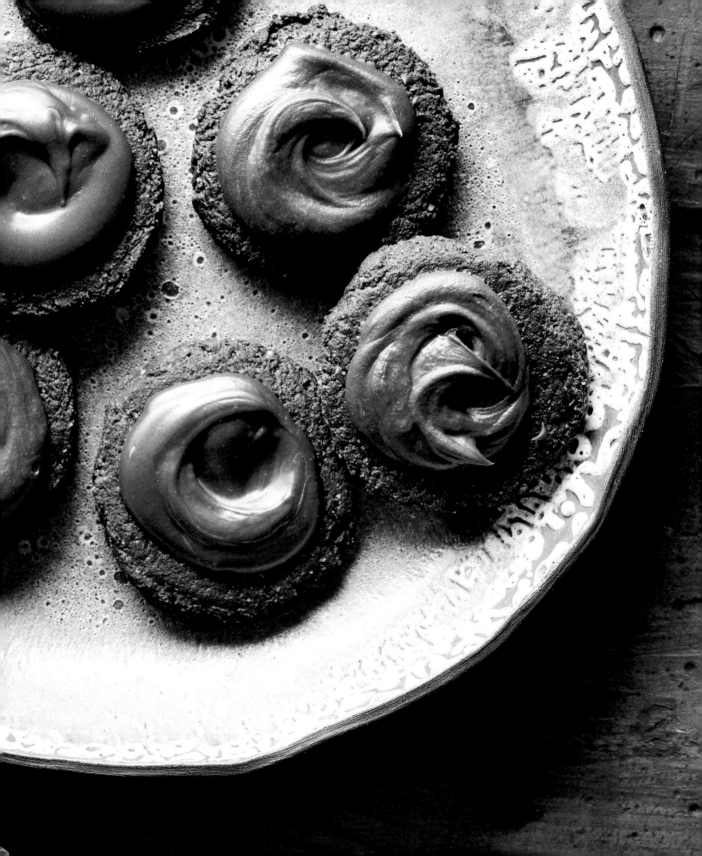

POPULAR KETO SWEETENER BLENDS

SWEETENER	BLEND
Lakanto	Blend of monkfruit and erythritol
Wholesome Provisions	Blend of allulose, monkfruit, and stevia
Swerve	Blend of erythritol and prebiotic oligosaccharides (from root vegetables)
Pyure Organic Stevia	Blend of erythritol, stevia, and fruit juice concentrate
Sukrin Gold	Blend of erythritol, steviol, glycosides (stevia), malt extract, tagatose
Xylitol	Pure xylitol
Allulose	Pure allulose
BochaSweet	Kabocha squash extract

EGG SUBSTITUTES

Flaxseed	1 tablespoon ground flaxseed + 3 tablespoons water = 1 large egg. Allow to set for 3 to 5 minutes to thicken.
Chia seed	1 tablespoon ground chia seeds + 3 tablespoons water = 1 large egg. Allow to set for 15 to 20 minutes to thicken.
Yogurt	¼ cup plain yogurt = 1 large egg
Arrowroot powder	2 tablespoons arrowroot powder + 3 tablespoons water = 1 large egg
Nut butter	3 tablespoons nut butter = 1 large egg
Avocado	¼ cup avocado puree = 1 large egg
Gelatin (unflavored)	For the equivalent of 1 egg: Dissolve 1 tablespoon unflavored gelatin in 1 tablespoon cold water, then add 2 tablespoons boiling water and mix until frothy.
Pumpkin Puree	¼ cup pumpkin puree = 1 large egg
Vinegar and baking soda	For the equivalent of 1 egg: Mix 1 teaspoon baking soda with 1 tablespoon apple cider vinegar.
Sour cream	1½ tablespoons sour cream whisked until light = 1 large egg
Cream cheese	¼ cup cream cheese = 1 large egg

DAIRY SUBSTITUTES

	TASTE	TEXTURE
Almond milk	Nutty	Thin, watery
Coconut milk	Strong coconut flavor	Fatty, thicker
Cashew milk	Mild	Thicker
Flax milk	Mild	Thin, watery
Pea milk	Slight protein aftertaste	Thicker

Additional Notes

- Nut butters can be used as a replacement for butter or fats.
- Nutritional yeast can be used as a replacement for cheese.
- Coconut oil can be used as a replacement for butter. (You can buy butter-flavored coconut oil.)
- Mashed avocado can be used as a replacement for butter.
- Unflavored and unsweetened nut milk yogurt and coconut yogurt can be used as a replacement for milk-based yogurt.

CHOOSING WHAT TO EAT AT A RESTAURANT

- Look for a restaurant that serves quality proteins.
- Choose a protein without a fried coating.
- Order without the sauce or with the sauce on the side.
- Add a side salad or vegetable.
- Look for bunless or lettuce-wrapped burgers.
- Order tacos without the shells. Or try a taco salad.
- Select pizza without the crust or cauliflower crust if it's keto approved.
- Try a sausage, egg, and cheese breakfast biscuit, minus the biscuit.
- Choose meat and a veggie. At a Mexican restaurant, you can ask for avocado or guacamole.
- Skip the chips and queso. Queso or cheese dip made in a restaurant has more than cheese in it. Most are made with flour, which you want to avoid.
- Review the menu online before you head to your favorite restaurant and plan your meals accordingly. You don't want to get there and be disappointed to find very little that you can actually eat.
- Don't be afraid to tell your waiter that you are trying to restrict carbohydrates and sugar. More often than not, they can help you.

EQUIPMENT AND INGREDIENTS

Here are the equipment and ingredients that will make your journey to keto easier.

Helpful Kitchen Tools

- Air fryer or toaster oven
- Baking dish
- Baking sheet
- Blender
- Bundt pan and 4-inch mini Bundt pans
- Cake pan and 3-inch mini cake pans
- Cast-iron skillet, 12-inch
- Cheese grater
- Cookie scoop
- Cutting boards: one for meat and one for vegetables
- Doughnut pan
- Food processor
- Frying pan
- Griddle
- Hand mixer
- Ice cream scoop, 3-tablespoon capacity
- Instant Pot or Ninja Foodi
- Knives, full set
- Lemon squeezer
- Loaf pan and mini loaf pans
- Microwave oven
- Mixing bowls: small, medium, and large
- Muffin tin
- Parchment paper
- Pie pan, 8-inch
- Pizza cutter
- Rolling pin
- Saucepan
- Silicone mats
- Soup pot
- Spatulas: metal and rubber
- Spiralizer
- Springform pan
- Tongs
- Waffle maker and mini waffle maker
- Wire rack

Approved Keto Ingredients

BASIC FLAVORINGS AND EXTRACTS

Flavorings tend to be more concentrated than extracts. For guidance, 1 teaspoon extract is equal to 4 to 5 drops of flavoring. I really like the LorAnn brand flavorings and emulsions or the One on One Flavors (OOOF) concentrates for keto baking. Both of these brands can be purchased on Amazon. I use the flavors below frequently in my baking.

- Almond extract
- Apple flavoring
- Banana flavoring
- Cake batter flavoring
- Caramel flavoring
- Carrot cake flavoring
- Cookie dough flavoring
- Cornbread flavoring
- Cream cheese flavoring
- Key lime extract
- Lemon extract or juice
- Peppermint extract
- Pineapple flavoring
- Raspberry flavoring
- Vanilla extract

BASIC SEASONINGS

- All Seasoning Spice (page 274)
- Chives, dried
- Cinnamon, ground
- Cocoa powder, unsweetened
- Cream of tartar
- Dill weed, dried
- Everything bagel seasoning
- Garlic powder
- Italian seasoning
- Lemon pepper seasoning
- McCormick's Montreal Steak seasoning
- Mustard, dry
- Nutmeg
- Old Bay seasoning
- Onion powder
- Oregano, dried
- Paprika (or smoked paprika)
- Parsley, dried
- Pepper, black
- Pepper, cayenne
- Pork panko or crushed pork rinds
- Pumpkin pie spice
- Ranch seasoning or Homemade Dry Ranch Seasoning (page 278)
- Redmond Real Salt organic season salt
- Rosemary, dried
- Salt, pink Himalayan
- Thyme, dried
- Taco Seasoning (page 275)

THICKENERS

- Chia seeds
- Cream, heavy whipping
- Cream cheese
- Guar gum
- Mayonnaise
- Nutritional yeast flakes
- Psyllium husk
- Sour cream
- Xanthan gum

FLOURS

- Almond flour, blanched
- Coconut flour
- Oat fiber (not oat flour)
- Pecan flour
- Pumpkin seed flour
- Sunflower seed flour
- Walnut flour

HEALTHY FATS

- Avocado
- Avocado oil
- Bacon grease
- Beef tallow
- Butter
- Chocolate chips: Lily's stevia-sweetened or ChocZero
- Coconut butter
- Coconut oil
- Ghee
- Lard
- Mayonnaise
- MCT oil
- Olive oil, extra-virgin
- Olives
- Sesame oil

PROTEINS

- Bacon (no-sugar-added and nitrite-free)
- Beef, ground
- Beef jerky (no-sugar-added)
- Beef ribs
- Beef roast
- Bone broth
- Bratwurst
- Chicken (dark cuts with the skin on)
- Collagen peptides, unflavored
- Duck
- Eggs
- Fish (bass, carp, flounder, halibut, mackerel, salmon, sardines, trout, tuna)
- Goose
- Ham
- Hot dogs (uncured)
- Kielbasa
- Pepperoni
- Pheasant
- Pork chops
- Pork ribs
- Pork rinds

- Pork roast
- Quail
- Salami
- Sausage
- Shellfish (crab meat, mussels, oysters, scallops, shrimp)
- Steak
- Turkey
- Veal

NUTS AND SEEDS

- Almonds
- Brazil nuts
- Cashews
- Chia seeds
- Flaxseeds
- Hazelnuts
- Hemp seeds
- Macadamia nuts
- Peanuts
- Pecans
- Pine nuts
- Pistachios
- Pumpkin seeds
- Sesame seeds
- Sunflower seeds
- Walnuts

HEALTHY CARBOHYDRATES

- Artichokes
- Arugula
- Asparagus
- Berries: blackberries, blueberries, raspberries, and strawberries
- Bok choy
- Broccoli
- Brussels sprouts
- Cabbage
- Cauliflower
- Celery
- Chicory greens
- Cranberries
- Cucumbers
- Eggplant
- Garlic
- Green beans
- Jicama
- Kale
- Leeks
- Lemons
- Lettuce
- Limes
- Mushrooms
- Okra
- Onions
- Peppers
- Pumpkin
- Radishes
- Rhubarb
- Scallions
- Shallots
- Snow peas
- Spinach
- Squash, spaghetti
- Tomatoes
- Watercress
- Zucchini

EASY SWAP OUTS

INSTEAD OF	EAT
Potatoes	Radishes
Bread	Lettuce wraps or cheese bread
Hamburger buns	Fluffy White Bread (page 171)
Hot dog buns	Fluffy White Bread (page 171)
Potato chips	Crispy Baked Cheese Chips (page 66)
Noodles or spaghetti	Cauliflower noodles, shirataki (miracle or konjac) noodles or spiralized zucchini
French fries	Rutabaga Fries (page 140) or Cheese-Crusted Zucchini Fries (page 138)
Crispy taco shells	Fried or baked cheese
Apples	Jicama, zucchini, Chayote Applesauce (page 245) or Chayote Compote (page 280)

ABOUT THE RECIPES

The recipes in the book are all baked, mostly in the oven, with a whole chapter on foil packs, one of my favorite ways to bake. But I've also included some recipes for chaffles, which have become super popular in the keto world and are "baked" in a waffle maker. Every recipe has nutritional information, so you'll be able to figure out the right balance of macronutrients.

Total Carbs vs. Net Carbs

The nutritional values in the book indicate total carbs. To calculate net carbs use this formula: Total Carbs—Fiber = Net Carbs.

Skip the Takeout

Sticking to a keto diet when dining can be challenging. Sit-down restaurants don't mention every ingredient in a dish on their menus and fast food is filled with unwanted ingredients and additives. So I have a whole chapter devoted to recipes for the food you think you can't eat, like pizza, fries, tacos, chicken Parmesan, and so much more.

Foil Pack Dinners

I love baking dinners via the en papillote method, which is when you wrap up ingredients in aluminum foil or parchment paper and bake in the oven. This technique will steam your food and keep it moist, plus you'll have fewer pans to wash.

If you use parchment paper, make sure you cut a sheet large enough to hold your food with a couple of extra inches that you can use to fold over and seal the package. I like using aluminum foil because it's easier to seal.

Making dinners this way is easy and fast. And if you are making dinner for a family of four, you can create a foil pack for each person using their favorite ingredients.

Chaffles and Waffles

What is a chaffle? It's a waffle made with cheese instead of flour. Cheese + Waffle = Chaffle! Some of the recipes scattered throughout the book are savory and are usually made with mozzarella cheese. Other recipes are sweet and use cream cheese as the base. There are some more traditional waffles as well, though they are made with alternative flours, like almond flour and coconut flour. All you really need to know is that they are all keto friendly.

Making keto treats in a waffle maker has become quite popular and even more so now that there is a new mini waffle maker that has hit the market and taken the keto community by storm. I love it because each mini waffle is one perfect serving. But never fear, you can use a regular waffle maker too.

I have included a few recipes that are definitely worth trying like the Pizza Chaffles (page 134), BLT Chaffle Sandwich (page 120), Chaffle Churros (page 209), and the incredible Birthday Chaffle Cake (page 229). No more breadless sandwiches or bunless burgers—make a chaffle!

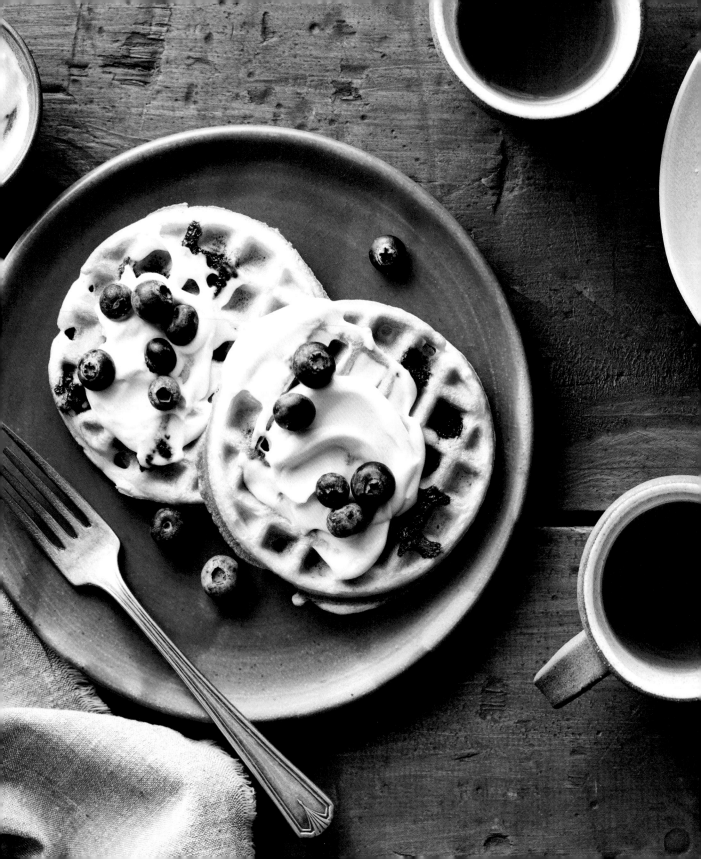

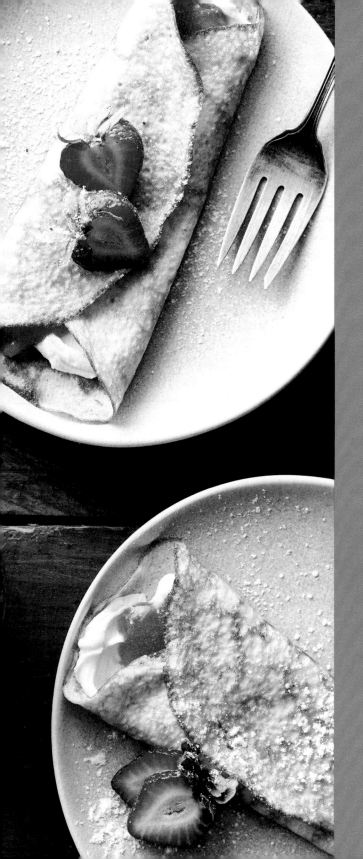

BREAKFAST

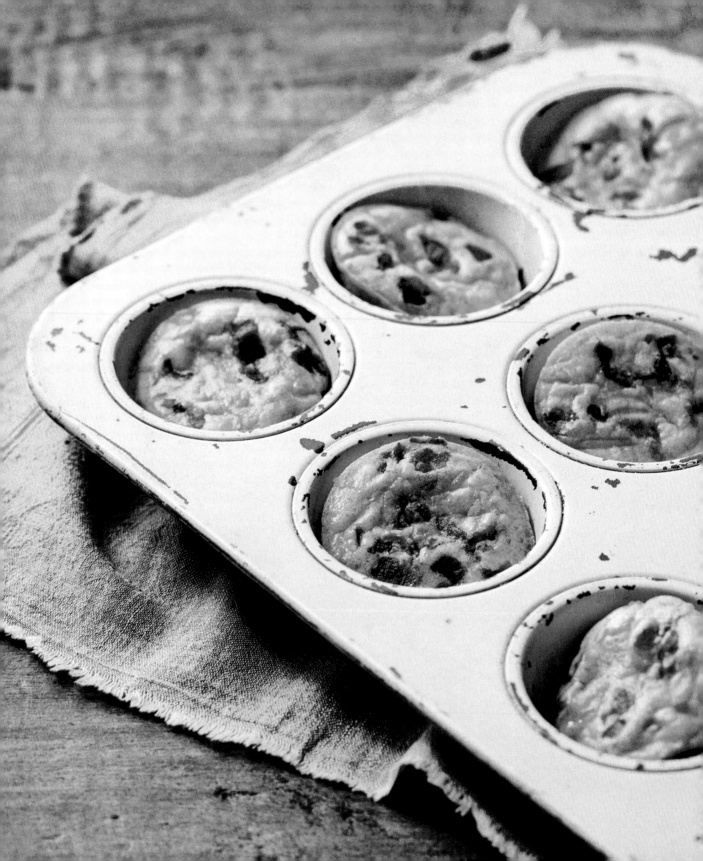

BACON AND CHEESE EGG BITES

8 large eggs

½ cup full-fat cottage
cheese

4 ounces shredded cheddar
cheese

6 slices Makin' Bacon
(page 270)

1 teaspoon pink
Himalayan salt

2 teaspoons Tabasco sauce
or Frank's RedHot hot sauce

MAKES 12 EGG BITES (12 SERVINGS)

What sets this recipe apart from other similar recipes is cottage cheese, which really gives the egg bites the perfect texture. Cream cheese is a fine substitute, but note that the nutritional values will change. Hot sauce contributes a kick of spice. The key to the recipe is to avoid overcooking, which will dry them out. To speed things up, I often buy already cooked bacon from Costco, or I make a batch of Makin' Bacon ahead of time.

PREHEAT the oven to 350°F. Spray a 12-cup muffin tin or 12 silicone muffin molds with cooking spray.

COMBINE the eggs, cottage cheese, cheddar cheese, bacon, salt, and Tabasco in a blender and blend on high for 20 to 30 seconds, until completely combined.

POUR the mixture equally into the prepared muffin tin. Bake for 10 to 12 minutes, until the egg bites are fully cooked.

WHILE they are still warm, remove the egg bites by running a knife around the edges of each one to loosen them from the sides of the muffin tin. They tend to stick more as they cool.

LEFTOVERS can be wrapped in a paper towel, placed in a zip-top bag, and refrigerated for 5 days. Reheat for 20 to 30 seconds in a microwave or eat them cold on the go.

NUTRITIONAL INFO (PER SERVING)
CALORIES 152, **FAT** 12.1g, **PROTEIN** 9.1g, **CARBS** 1.2g, **FIBER** 0g

ROASTED TURNIP HASH BROWNS WITH BAKED EGGS

3 medium turnips, diced

¼ cup extra-virgin olive oil

SPICY ROASTED
  TURNIPS

1 teaspoon smoked paprika

1 teaspoon salt

½ teaspoon garlic powder

½ teaspoon onion powder

½ teaspoon black pepper

1 teaspoon Tabasco sauce,
  optional

HERB ROASTED TURNIPS

1 teaspoon dried rosemary

1 teaspoon salt

¼ teaspoon garlic powder

¼ teaspoon onion powder

½ teaspoon black pepper

4 large eggs

MAKES 4 SERVINGS

Get ready to fall in love with turnips after eating these hash browns. Oven roasting brings out the natural sugars in the turnips and makes them mighty delicious. Take your pick from the spicy or nonspicy versions below. For the spicy turnips, if you don't have smoked paprika, go ahead and use chili powder.

PREHEAT the oven to 350°F. Line a baking sheet with parchment paper or a silicone mat.

IN a medium bowl, mix together the diced turnips and olive oil. Then add the spices for spicy or herb and mix well.

PLACE the turnips on the prepared baking sheet and bake for 20 to 25 minutes, until golden and tender.

MAKE four indentations in the hash browns and crack an egg into each one. Roast for an additional 10 minutes, or until the eggs are cooked to your preference.

NUTRITIONAL INFO (PER SERVING)
CALORIES 152, **FAT** 14.2g, **PROTEIN** 1.1g, **CARBS** 7.3g, **FIBER** 2.1g

CRUSTLESS CHORIZO BREAKFAST BAKE

1 tablespoon extra-virgin olive oil

½ cup diced onion

½ cup diced green bell pepper

½ cup diced red bell pepper

1 pound Mexican chorizo sausage

8 large eggs

½ cup heavy whipping cream

1 tablespoon sriracha

½ teaspoon chili powder

½ teaspoon salt

½ teaspoon black pepper

2 cups shredded cheddar cheese

MAKES 10 SERVINGS

If you are in the mood for a breakfast idea with Mexican flare, this recipe will hit the spot. It makes a delicious brunch dish for company and it warms up nicely the next day too.

PREHEAT the oven to 350°F. Have a 3-quart baking dish ready.

IN a medium skillet over medium heat, heat the oil. Add the onion and red and green bell pepper and cook, stirring, until soft, about 5 minutes. Add the chorizo and cook, breaking it up with a wooden spoon, until browned. Drain and discard the fat.

IN a large bowl, whisk together the eggs, cream, sriracha, chili powder, salt, and pepper until frothy. Add the chorizo mixture to the egg mixture and fold in the cheese.

TRANSFER the mixture to the baking dish and bake for 40 minutes, or until the eggs are set and fully cooked. Serve hot.

NUTRITIONAL INFO (PER SERVING)
CALORIES 305, **FAT** 24.8g, **PROTEIN** 16.4g, **CARBS** 3.2g, **FIBER** 0.5g

BACON-SPINACH-FETA BREAKFAST PINWHEELS

FILLING

3 tablespoons extra-virgin olive oil

8 ounces fresh spinach, chopped

1 teaspoon minced garlic

1 teaspoon salt

DOUGH

2 cups shredded part-skim low-moisture mozzarella cheese

2 ounces Alouette garlic and herbs soft spreadable cheese

1 large egg

½ cup blanched almond flour

3 ounces Alouette garlic and herbs soft spreadable cheese

4 slices Makin' Bacon (page 270), crumbled

2 ounces feta, crumbled

MAKES 12 PINWHEELS (6 SERVINGS)

This recipe was inspired by a low-carb pizza crust recipe, with an added twist of savory ingredients to make a satisfying breakfast that is sure to impress!

PREHEAT the oven to 350°F. Have a 12-cup muffin tin ready. Have two large sheets of parchment paper ready.

FOR THE FILLING

IN a large skillet over medium heat, heat the oil. Add the spinach, garlic, and salt and cook, stirring frequently, until the spinach is tender, about 3 minutes. Set aside to cool.

FOR THE DOUGH

IN a microwave-safe bowl, mix together the mozzarella cheese and Alouette cheese and heat in the microwave for about 1 minute, until the mozzarella has melted. Add the egg and almond flour and mix together until it forms a soft dough.

TRANSFER the dough onto one sheet of parchment paper and knead until smooth. If the dough becomes stiff, heat it for another 15 seconds in the microwave, or until soft. Place the second sheet of parchment paper on top of the dough. Using a rolling pin, roll out the dough into an 11- by 14-inch rectangle, about ¼ inch thick.

TO ASSEMBLE THE PINWHEELS

SPREAD the Alouette cheese over the dough, leaving about 1 inch of dough on all sides. Arrange the spinach over the cheese and sprinkle with the bacon and feta cheese. Starting at the short end, roll up the dough.

(continued)

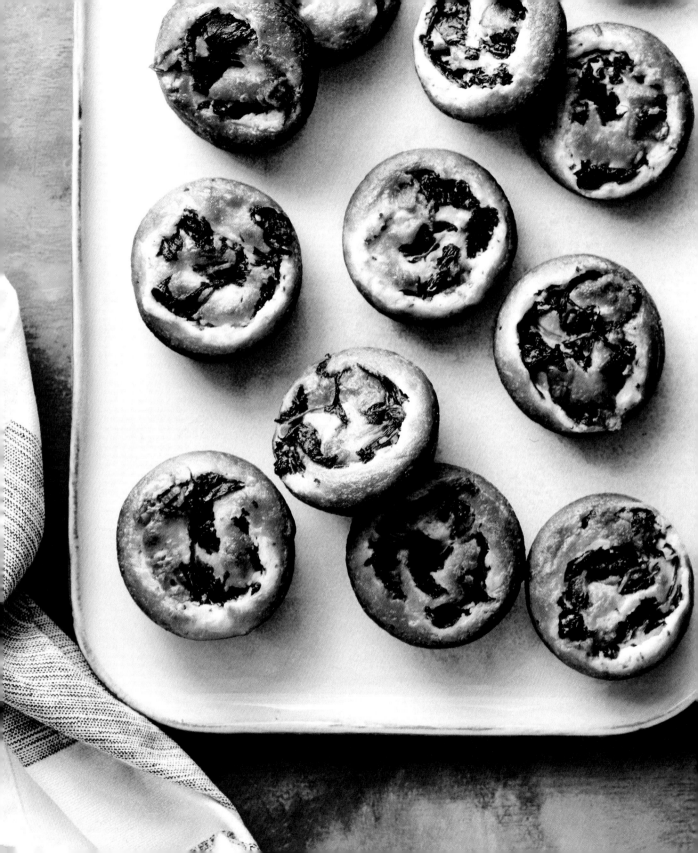

CUTTING slices with a knife will flatten the dough, so instead I use string: Cut 12 even slices by placing the string under the dough, crisscrossing it over the top, and pulling both ends of the string to make a clean cut.

PLACE each slice in a muffin cup and bake for 15 to 18 minutes, until golden brown. Serve warm.

STORE leftovers in a covered container in the refrigerator for up to 4 days. Reheat in the microwave for about 20 seconds. They are perfect for a quick breakfast.

NUTRITIONAL INFO (PER SERVING)
CALORIES 170, **FAT** 7.9g, **PROTEIN** 15g, **CARBS** 9.7g, **FIBER** 4.7g

BREAKFAST PIZZA

DOUGH

1½ cups shredded part-skim low-moisture mozzarella cheese

2 ounces cream cheese, at room temperature

1 large egg

¾ cup blanched almond flour

TOPPING

1 tablespoon butter, melted

1 tablespoon Italian seasoning

6 large eggs

1 tablespoon heavy whipping cream

1 teaspoon salt

½ teaspoon black pepper

1 tablespoon extra-virgin olive oil

1 cup shredded Monterey Jack cheese

½ cup shredded cheddar cheese

4 slices Makin' Bacon (page 270), crumbled

MAKES 8 SERVINGS

I've taken pizza and turned it into your new favorite morning repast. This hearty combination of ingredients will load you up with energy and keep you full for hours.

PREHEAT the oven to 350°F. Line a baking sheet with parchment paper or a silicone mat. Have two sheets of parchment paper ready.

FOR THE DOUGH

IN a microwave-safe bowl, mix together the mozzarella cheese and cream cheese. Heat in the microwave for 1 minute, or until the mozzarella has melted. Add the egg and almond flour and mix until fully combined.

TRANSFER the dough to one sheet of parchment paper and knead until smooth. Place the second sheet of parchment paper over the top and, using a rolling pin, roll it out into a large round about ¼ inch thick. Transfer the dough to the baking sheet and bake for 12 to 15 minutes, until slightly browned.

FOR THE TOPPING

SPREAD the melted butter onto the crust and sprinkle with the Italian seasoning.

IN a medium bowl, whisk together the eggs, cream, salt, and pepper. In a medium skillet over medium heat, heat the olive oil. Pour in the egg mixture and cook, stirring occasionally, until the mixture is no longer wet, 5 to 7 minutes.

SPREAD the egg mixture evenly over the pizza crust. Sprinkle with the Monterey Jack, cheddar, and bacon. Bake for 5 to 8 minutes, or just until the cheese has melted. Cut into 8 slices and serve.

NUTRITIONAL INFO (PER SERVING)
CALORIES 344, **FAT** 24.2g, **PROTEIN** 20.2g, **CARBS** 4.2g, **FIBER** 0.8g

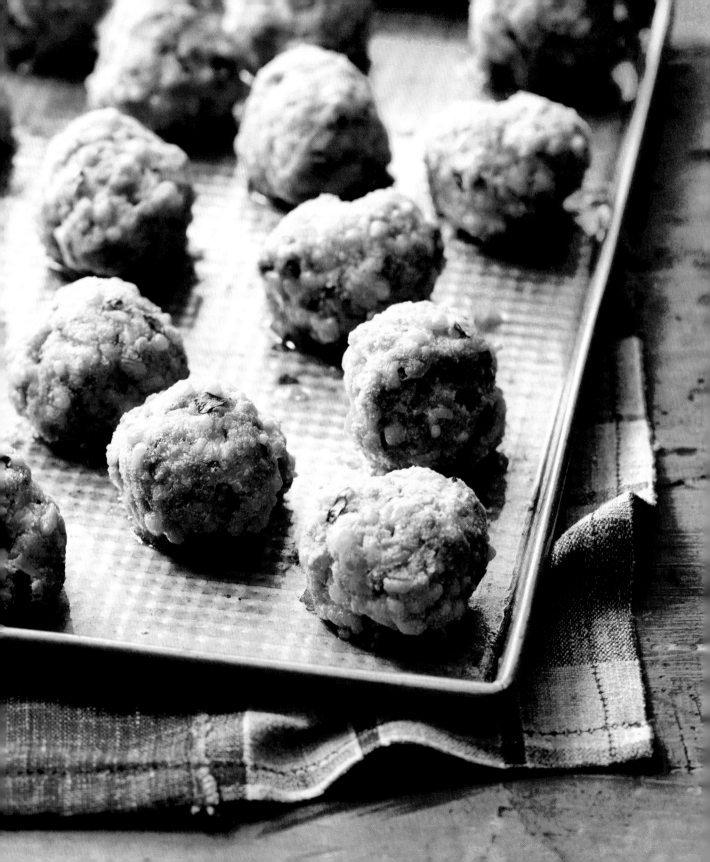

SAUSAGE BALLS

1 pound ground pork

2 cups shredded cheddar
cheese

¾ cup blanched almond flour

¼ cup coconut flour

1 tablespoon chopped
fresh parsley

1 tablespoon cream cheese,
at room temperature

1 teaspoon onion powder

1 teaspoon salt

½ teaspoon dry mustard

½ teaspoon paprika

MAKES 12 BALLS

Although these are great for breakfast, they make an excellent party appetizer too.

PREHEAT the oven to 350°F. Line a baking sheet with parchment paper or a silicone mat.

IN a medium bowl, combine all the ingredients, using your hands to incorporate the ingredients until they come together.

FORM the mixture into balls, using an ice cream scoop to make 12 large sausage balls or a cookie scoop to make 24 small sausage balls. Place the balls on the baking sheet.

BAKE large sausage balls for 30 minutes or small ones for 20 minutes, or until golden brown and fully cooked.

Note: *You can make the sausage balls ahead of time. Simply form as instructed and place them on the baking sheet. Instead of baking, cover the sheet with aluminum foil and freeze for at least 3 hours. Transfer the frozen sausage balls to a zip-top bag and store in the freezer for up to 4 months. When you are ready to cook them, defrost the sausage balls for 15 to 20 minutes, then bake as instructed.*

NUTRITIONAL INFO (PER SERVING)
CALORIES 154, **FAT** 10.2g, **PROTEIN** 7g, **CARBS** 3.9g, **FIBER** 1.2g

BLUEBERRY–CREAM CHEESE DANISH

BLUEBERRY FILLING

1 cup fresh blueberries

3 tablespoons monkfruit powdered sweetener

2 tablespoons lemon juice

1 teaspoon vanilla extract

¼ teaspoon liquid stevia

½ teaspoon xanthan gum

DOUGH

2 cups shredded part-skim low-moisture mozzarella cheese

2 ounces cream cheese, at room temperature

½ cup blanched almond flour

¼ cup coconut flour

2 tablespoons monkfruit powdered sweetener

½ teaspoon LorAnn buttery sweet dough bakery emulsion

CREAM CHEESE FILLING

6 ounces cream cheese, at room temperature

¼ cup monkfruit powdered sweetener

1 teaspoon vanilla extract

1 teaspoon lemon juice

MAKES 6 LARGE DANISH (12 SERVINGS)

This is what I make for breakfast when we need a sweet treat. It's impressive enough to serve to guests too. You can make the pastries ahead of time as they taste amazing hot out of the oven, cold, or warmed up in the microwave for about 10 seconds.

PREHEAT the oven to 350°F. Line a baking sheet with parchment paper or a silicone mat. Have a second sheet of parchment paper ready.

FOR THE BLUEBERRY FILLING

IN a medium saucepan over medium heat, mix together the blueberries, sweetener, lemon juice, vanilla, and stevia. Bring to a simmer and cook, stirring, until the sauce thickens, 5 to 7 minutes. Sprinkle with the xanthan gum and mix until fully combined. Set aside to cool.

FOR THE DOUGH

IN a small microwave-safe bowl, mix together the mozzarella cheese and cream cheese and heat in the microwave oven for 1 minute, or until the cheese has completely melted. Add the almond flour, coconut flour, sweetener, and bakery emulsion and stir to combine.

TRANSFER the dough to the parchment paper and knead until it fully comes together. Divide the dough into six equal pieces. If the dough becomes stiff, heat it for 15 seconds in the microwave, or until soft. Shape each piece of dough into a 3-inch round with raised edges (to hold the filling in) and transfer to the lined baking sheet. Set aside.

(ingredients and recipe continued)

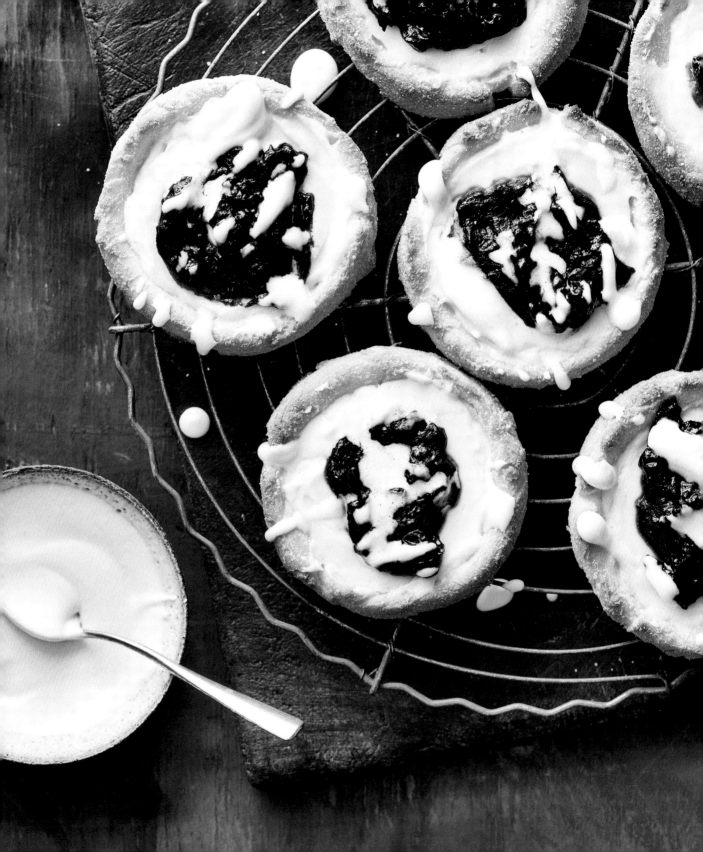

GLAZE

¼ cup heavy whipping cream

2 tablespoons monkfruit powdered sweetener

FOR THE CREAM CHEESE FILLING

IN a small bowl using a hand mixer, beat the cream cheese, sweetener, vanilla, and lemon juice until smooth, about 2 minutes. Spoon the filling equally onto the six dough rounds. Spoon 2 tablespoons of blueberry filling over the cream cheese filling.

BAKE for 20 to 25 minutes, until the edges of the dough are golden brown. Transfer the Danish to a wire rack to cool.

FOR THE GLAZE

IN a small bowl using a hand mixer, beat the cream, sweetener, and ½ teaspoon water until smooth. Drizzle the glaze over each Danish, cut each in half, and serve.

NUTRITIONAL INFO (PER ½ DANISH)
CALORIES 165, **FAT** 11.4g, **PROTEIN** 5.9g, **CARBS** 9.1g, **FIBER** 1.3g

DUTCH BABY PANCAKE

1 tablespoon extra-virgin
olive oil

3 large eggs

2 ounces cream cheese, at
room temperature

2 tablespoons butter, melted

1 teaspoon vanilla extract

1 teaspoon Swerve
confectioners' sweetener

½ teaspoon baking powder

MAKES 2 SERVINGS

I should call this a lazy Dutch baby pancake because the sides don't rise as high as a regular Dutch baby—but who cares because it tastes absolutely amazing. Top it with your favorite sugar-free syrup and dust a bit of extra confectioners' sugar over the top for a delightful breakfast that will please everyone.

PREHEAT the oven to 350°F.

POUR 1 tablespoon of olive oil into a 10-inch cast-iron skillet. Place the skillet in the oven to warm up while you make the batter.

COMBINE the eggs, cream cheese, butter, vanilla, sweetener, and baking powder in a blender and blend on high for about 2 minutes, or until the batter is completely smooth.

POUR the batter into the preheated cast-iron skillet and bake for 5 minutes, or until the batter is not jiggly. Serve warm.

NUTRITIONAL INFO (PER SERVING)
CALORIES 218, **FAT** 19g, **PROTEIN** 8.9g, **CARBS** 2.3g, **FIBER** 2.1g

CINNAMON FRENCH TOAST

2 large eggs

1 tablespoon heavy whipping cream

½ teaspoon ground cinnamon

½ teaspoon vanilla extract

1 teaspoon extra-virgin olive oil

4 slices Fluffy White Bread (page 171)

Sugar-free maple syrup, optional

MAKES 4 SERVINGS

When I have a bit of extra time and I want breakfast to be extra special, this is what I make. It's a festive dish to serve on holidays, and the cinnamon aroma as it bakes is delightful.

IN a small bowl, whisk the eggs until frothy. Add the cream, cinnamon, and vanilla and whisk until well combined.

IN a medium skillet over medium heat, heat the olive oil. Dip one slice of the bread into the egg mixture, making sure to coat both sides. Place the bread in the skillet and cook until golden brown, about 2 minutes on each side. Repeat with the rest of the bread.

SERVE immediately with syrup on the side, if using.

NUTRITIONAL INFO (PER SERVING)
CALORIES 258, **FAT** 16.5g, **PROTEIN** 12.4g, **CARBS** 4.8g, **FIBER** 0.7g

SWEET BREAKFAST CREPES

STRAWBERRY COMPOTE

1 cup chopped strawberries

¼ cup monkfruit powdered sweetener

2 tablespoons lemon juice

½ teaspoon xanthan gum

FILLING

4 ounces cream cheese, at room temperature

2 teaspoons monkfruit powdered sweetener

1 teaspoon heavy whipping cream

1 teaspoon vanilla extract

CREPES

4 large eggs

4 ounces cream cheese, at room temperature

1 tablespoon butter

2 teaspoons monkfruit powdered sweetener

1 teaspoon psyllium husk powder

1 teaspoon extra-virgin olive oil, plus more as needed

OPTIONAL TOPPINGS

Sliced strawberries

Monkfruit powdered sweetener

MAKES 6 SERVINGS

Crepes sound fancy, but they are actually pretty easy to make. The strawberry compote pairs perfectly with the cream cheese filling, making this tasty and healthy while keeping you full for hours.

FOR THE COMPOTE

IN a small saucepan over medium heat, mix together the strawberries, sweetener, and lemon juice. Cook, stirring, until the strawberries break down and turn into a thick sauce. Sprinkle in the xanthan gum and stir to combine. Set aside.

FOR THE FILLING

IN a medium bowl using a hand mixer, beat together the cream cheese, sweetener, cream, and vanilla until light and smooth. Set aside.

FOR THE CREPES

IN a medium bowl using a hand mixer, beat together the eggs, cream cheese, butter, sweetener, and psyllium husk powder until smooth.

IN a medium skillet over medium-high heat, heat the oil. Spoon about 2 tablespoons of batter onto the skillet, spread very thin, and cook until firm, 1 to 2 minutes. Using a wide spatula, flip the crepe and cook until just beginning to brown. Transfer to a plate. Repeat with the rest of the batter, adding oil to the skillet as needed to keep them from sticking.

(continued)

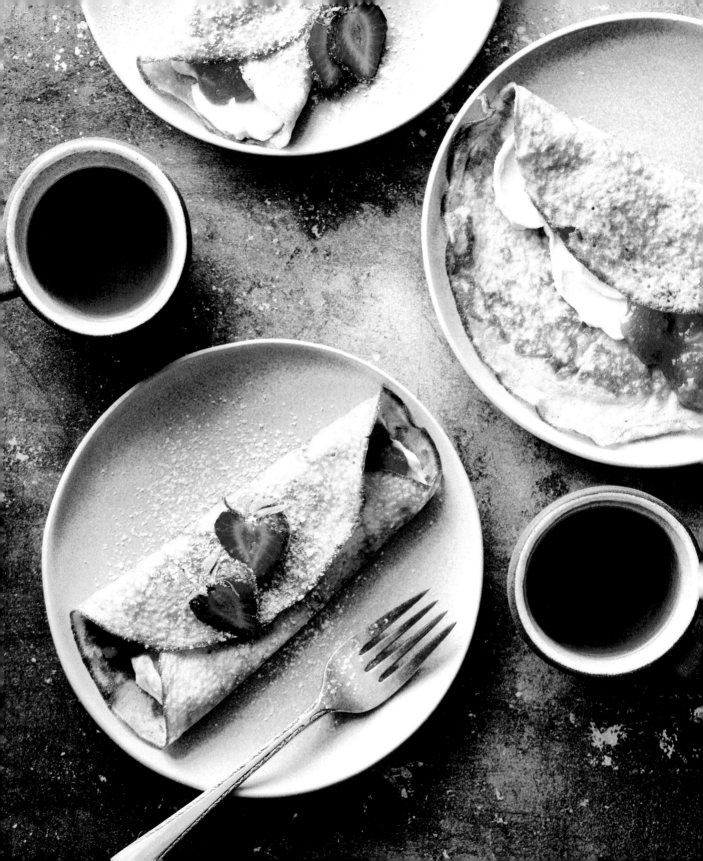

TO assemble, spread a crepe with the cream cheese filling and top with the strawberry compote. Roll up the crepe and place on a plate. Spoon more strawberry compote over the top and, if desired, top with sliced strawberries and powdered sweetener. Serve warm.

NUTRITIONAL INFO (PER SERVING)
CALORIES 217, **FAT** 19.1g, **PROTEIN** 6.7g, **CARBS** 7.8g, **FIBER** 0.7g

BLUEBERRY WAFFLES

1 large egg

3 tablespoons blanched
   almond flour

1 tablespoon cream cheese,
   at room temperature

¼ teaspoon baking powder

4 drops LorAnn Naturals
   blueberry flavoring, optional

5 or 6 fresh blueberries, plus
   more for topping

Monkfruit powdered
   sweetener, optional

OPTIONAL TOPPINGS
(PAGE 54)

MAKES 2 WAFFLES (1 SERVING)

I used a mini waffle maker to make these waffles. If you use a regular-size waffle maker the batter will fill it to make one large waffle.

PREHEAT a mini waffle maker according to the manufacturers' instructions.

IN a small bowl, whisk the egg. Add the almond flour, cream cheese, baking powder, and blueberry flavoring, if using, and whisk until smooth. Fold in the blueberries.

SPRAY the waffle maker with cooking spray. Spoon half of the batter into the waffle maker and cook until golden brown, 3 to 4 minutes. Repeat with the rest of the batter.

SERVE the waffle plain or topped with a dusting of monkfruit sweetener, or additional blueberries. You can also top with one of the toppings.

(continued)

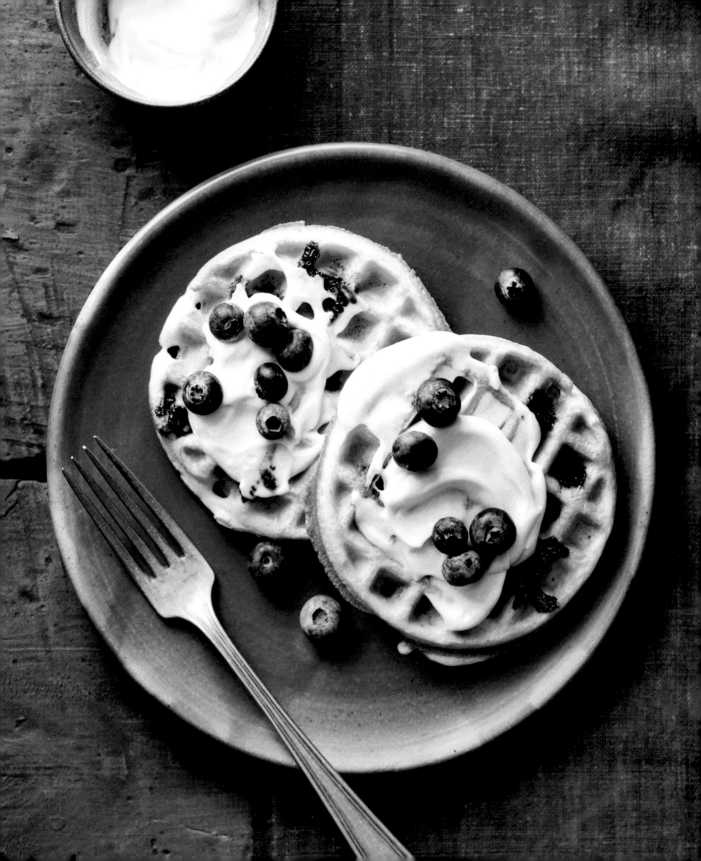

OPTIONAL TOPPINGS

GLAZE: Warm 1 tablespoon cream cheese in the microwave for 15 seconds, add 4 drops blueberry flavoring and 1 tablespoon monkfruit powdered sweetener, and stir until smooth. Spread over the warm waffles.

CREAM CHEESE FROSTING: Mix together 1 tablespoon cream cheese (at room temperature), 4 drops blueberry flavoring, 1 tablespoon butter (at room temperature), and 1 tablespoon monkfruit powdered sweetener until smooth. Spread over the warm waffles.

WHIPPED CREAM: Using a hand mixer, beat ¼ cup heavy whipping cream, ¼ teaspoon vanilla extract, and 1 teaspoon monkfruit powdered sweetener until peaks form. Dollop over the warm waffles.

NUTRITIONAL INFO (PER SERVING)
CALORIES 249, **FAT** 13.5g, **PROTEIN** 10.2g, **CARBS** 7.3g, **FIBER** 1g

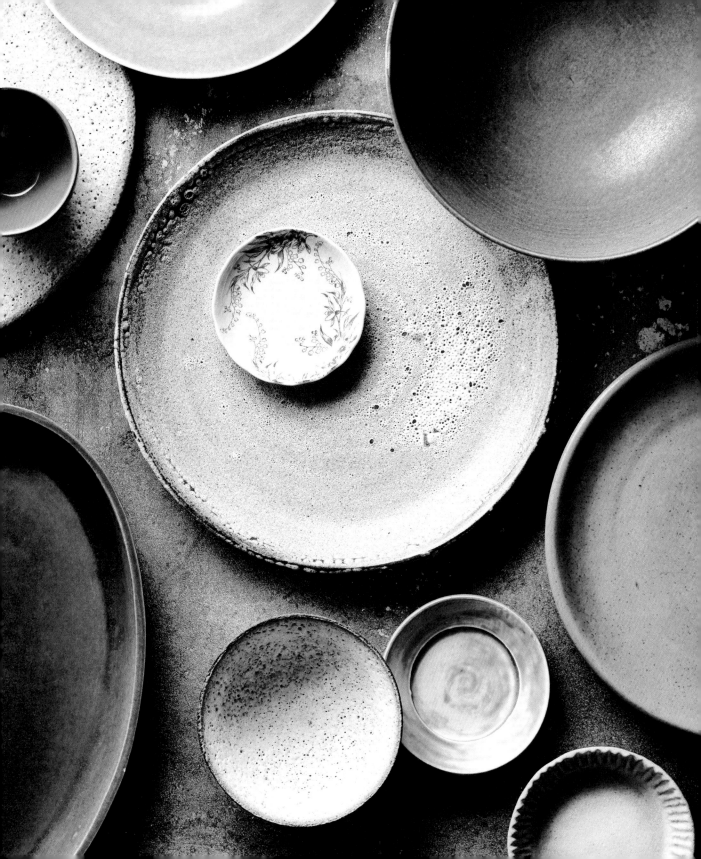

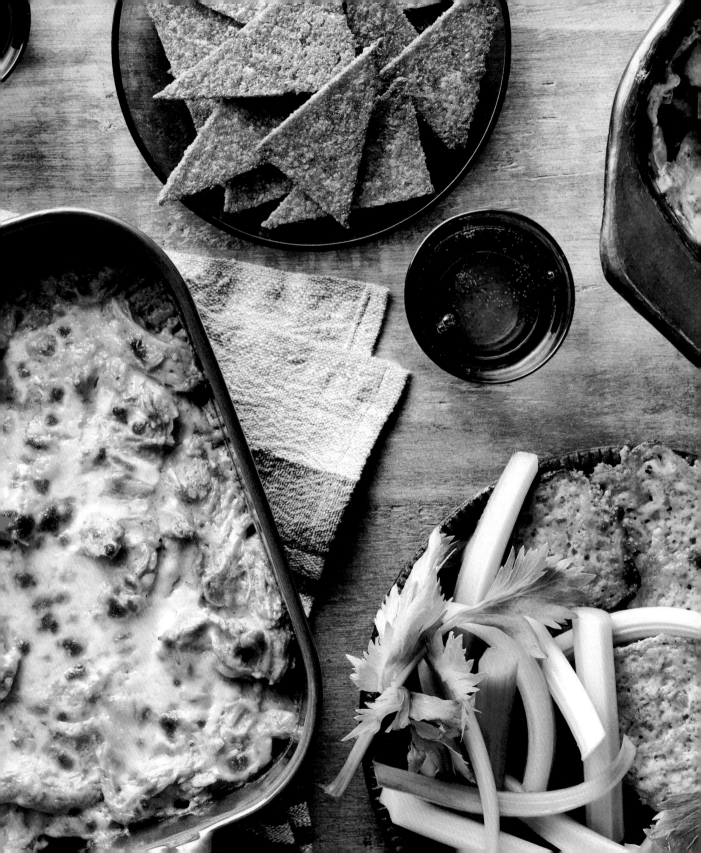

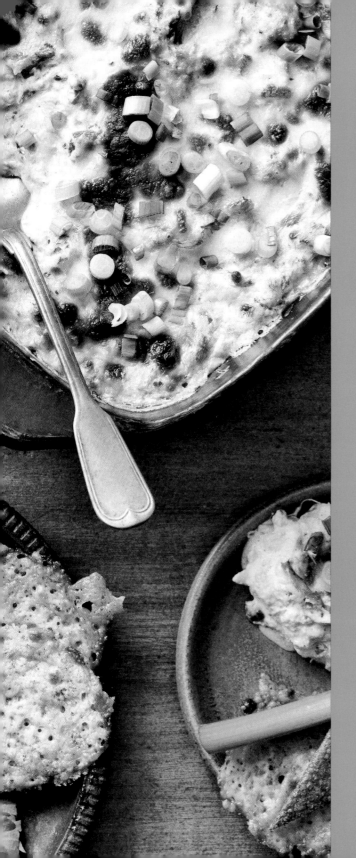

BAKED APPETIZERS

PIZZA BAGELS

2½ cups shredded part-skim low-moisture mozzarella cheese

3 tablespoons cream cheese, at room temperature

1¼ cups blanched almond flour

2 teaspoons baking powder

1 teaspoon Italian seasoning

½ teaspoon garlic powder

¼ teaspoon salt

1 large egg

¼ cup grated Parmesan cheese

¼ cup mini pepperoni slices

Fresh basil leaves, optional

MAKES 6 LARGE PIZZA BAGELS

If you need a fun snack or an appetizer for a party, you've come to the right place! These are pretty great on their own, or serve them with small bowls of Rao's marinara as a dipping sauce.

PREHEAT the oven to 375°F. Line a baking sheet with parchment paper or a silicone mat. Have a sheet of parchment paper ready.

IN a microwave-safe bowl, combine the mozzarella and cream cheese and heat on high for 1 to 1½ minutes, until the cheese has melted. Add the almond flour, baking powder, Italian seasoning, garlic powder, salt, and egg and stir to combine.

KNEAD the dough on the parchment paper until fully combined and no longer sticky. If the dough becomes too stiff, microwave for 30 seconds and continue to knead.

DIVIDE the dough into six equal pieces. Roll one piece into a 5-inch rope and press the ends together to form a ring. Be sure to leave a big enough opening in the center for the hole. Place the ring on the prepared baking sheet. Repeat with the rest of the dough.

SPRINKLE the top of the dough rings with Parmesan cheese, pepperoni slices, and basil, if using.

BAKE for 11 to 13 minutes, until golden brown. Transfer to a wire rack and let cool for about 5 minutes before cutting them horizontally.

NUTRITIONAL INFO (PER BAGEL)
CALORIES 298, **FAT** 15.5g, **PROTEIN** 14.6g, **CARBS** 9.5g, **FIBER** 1g

MEXICAN QUESO

4 ounces cream cheese, at room temperature

1 cup heavy whipping cream

1 cup shredded cheddar cheese

½ cup shredded Monterey Jack cheese

3 tablespoons butter

2 teaspoons Frank's RedHot hot sauce

½ teaspoon garlic powder

¼ teaspoon dry mustard

¼ teaspoon salt

¼ teaspoon black pepper

1 (10-ounce) can Ro*Tel diced tomatoes and green chilies

MAKES 6 SERVINGS

This is a wonderful recipe that does double-duty: It can be poured over your favorite vegetables or used as a dip with Rutabaga Fries (page 140), pork rinds, or your favorite raw veggies.

IN a saucepan over medium heat, mix together the cream cheese, cream, cheddar, Monterey Jack, butter, hot sauce, garlic powder, mustard, salt, and pepper until the cheese has melted and the mixture is smooth.

LOWER the heat to medium-low and simmer until the sauce thickens, 4 to 5 minutes. Add the Ro*Tel and stir until combined.

SERVE immediately or store in a covered container in the refrigerator for up to 1 week.

NUTRITIONAL INFO (PER SERVING)
CALORIES 325, **FAT** 30.2g, **PROTEIN** 9.9g, **CARBS** 4.3g, **FIBER** 0.4g

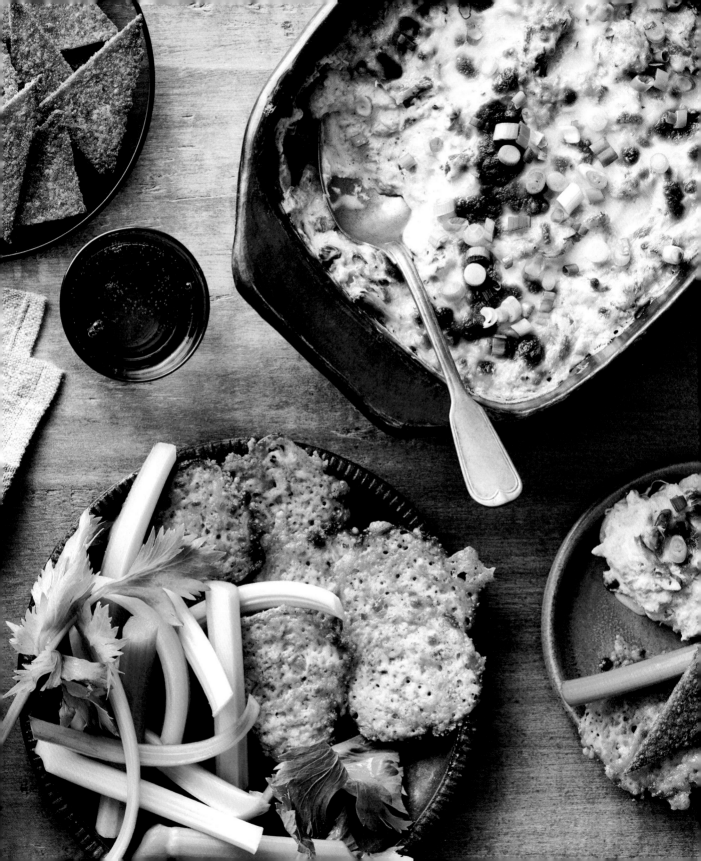

CRAB RANGOON DIP

2 cups (about 16 ounces) fresh crabmeat

8 ounces cream cheese, at room temperature

1 cup shredded part-skim low-moisture mozzarella cheese

Juice of ½ lemon

2 teaspoons mayonnaise

2 teaspoons coconut aminos

¼ teaspoon liquid stevia

¼ cup jarred diced pimientos, drained

1 tablespoon sliced green onions

½ teaspoon garlic powder

¼ teaspoon black pepper

Salt

OPTIONAL TOPPINGS

Chopped scallions, optional

MAKES 8 SERVINGS

This is a must-have appetizer for a party or for simply relaxing at home with the family. The low-carb, creamy, cheesy, hot dip—loaded with crab—goes well with celery sticks or other raw veggies. Bring this dip to a party and no one will ever know it's a healthy, keto friendly treat.

PREHEAT the oven to 350°F. Spray a 2½-quart baking dish with cooking spray.

IN a large bowl, mix together the crab, cream cheese, ½ cup of mozzarella, the lemon juice, mayonnaise, coconut aminos, stevia, pimientos, green onions, garlic powder, and pepper. Taste and season with salt. Transfer the mixture to the prepared baking dish and sprinkle the remaining ½ cup of mozzarella over the top.

BAKE for 20 minutes, or until the cheese has melted and is golden brown. Sprinkle with scallions, if using.

NUTRITIONAL INFO (PER SERVING)
CALORIES 214, **FAT** 13.7g, **PROTEIN** 18g, **CARBS** 5.1g, **FIBER** 0.3g

BUFFALO CHICKEN DIP

5 ounces cream cheese, at room temperature

½ cup mayonnaise

½ cup Frank's RedHot buffalo wings sauce

2 teaspoons minced garlic

½ teaspoon paprika

½ teaspoon salt

½ teaspoon black pepper

1 cup shredded part-skim low-moisture mozzarella cheese

20 ounces shredded cooked chicken

½ cup shredded Asiago cheese

Celery sticks, for dipping

Keto Chips (page 65), for dipping

MAKES 10 SERVINGS

Buy shredded cooked chicken or two (10-ounce) cans chicken at the grocery store or use leftover chicken for this dip. Serve it with celery sticks or pork rinds.

PREHEAT the oven to 375°F. Spray a 9-inch square baking dish with cooking spray.

IN a medium bowl using a hand mixer, beat the cream cheese, mayonnaise, buffalo sauce, garlic, paprika, salt, and pepper until smooth. Add ½ cup of the mozzarella and beat well. Add the chicken and mix with a spoon until fully combined. Transfer to the prepared baking dish and top with the remaining ½ cup mozzarella and the Asiago cheese.

BAKE for 20 minutes, or until the cheese is bubbly and golden brown. Serve warm with celery sticks or keto chips on the side for dipping.

NUTRITIONAL INFO (PER SERVING)
CALORIES 238, **FAT** 17.4g, **PROTEIN** 17.4g, **CARBS** 2.3g, **FIBER** 0.2g

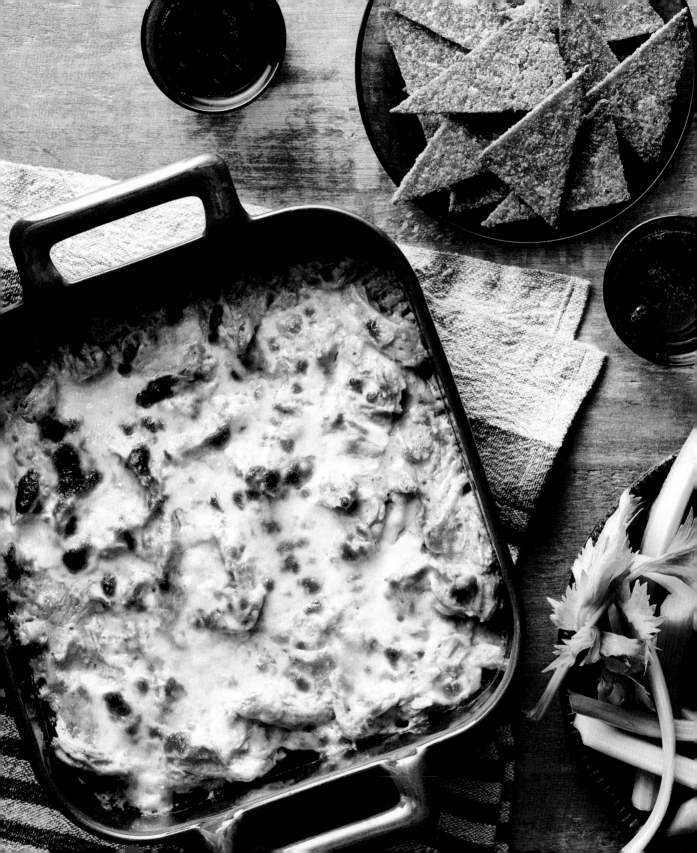

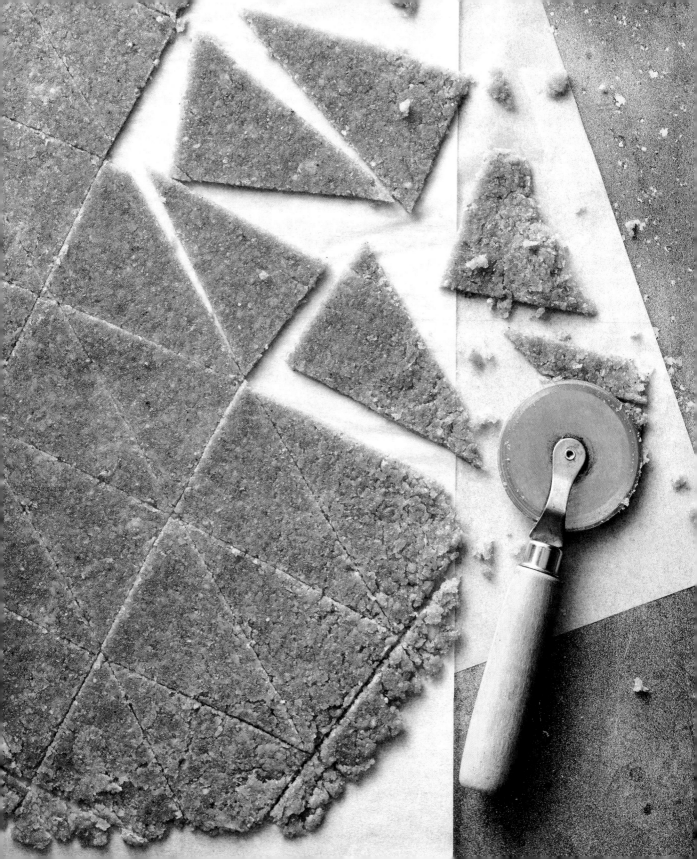

KETO CHIPS

½ cup shredded part-skim low-moisture mozzarella cheese

½ cup shredded Monterey Jack cheese

2 ounces cream cheese, at room temperature

2 cups pork panko or crushed pork rinds

1 large egg white

1 teaspoon salt

½ teaspoon paprika

¼ teaspoon garlic powder

¼ teaspoon onion powder

¼ teaspoon ground cumin

¼ teaspoon chili powder

MAKES 8 SERVINGS

This chip holds up when served with a hearty dip, so it's great for parties. I often eat them when I just want a clean snack as well. They taste amazing fresh out of the oven. Serve with any of the hearty dips in this chapter.

PREHEAT the oven to 450°F. Line a baking sheet with parchment paper or a silicone mat. Have two large sheets of parchment paper ready.

IN a large microwave-safe bowl, mix together the mozzarella, Monterey Jack, and cream cheese and heat in the microwave oven for 30 to 60 seconds, until completely melted. Add the pork panko, egg white, salt, paprika, garlic powder, onion powder, cumin, and chili powder and mix until fully combined. The dough will be somewhat sticky.

KNEAD the dough on one sheet of parchment paper until it comes together and is less sticky. Place the second piece of parchment over it. Using a rolling pin, roll the dough out as thin as you can. Using a pizza cutter, cut 2-inch triangles out of the dough and place them on the prepared baking sheet.

BAKE for 10 minutes, or until the chips are crispy and golden brown. Serve immediately. The chips are best eaten right away because they lose their crunch quickly.

NUTRITIONAL INFO (PER SERVING)
CALORIES 391, **FAT** 24.4g, **PROTEIN** 39.4g, **CARBS** 1.2g, **FIBER** 0.1g

CRISPY BAKED CHEESE CHIPS

½ cup shredded cheddar cheese

½ cup shredded part-skim low-moisture mozzarella cheese

½ cup grated Parmesan cheese

1 teaspoon All Seasoning Spice (page 274)

MAKES 4 SERVINGS (24 TOTAL CHIPS)

These pair well with any of the dips in this chapter. Try sprinkling with other seasonings or herbs. I like using Everything Bagel seasoning, which you can buy at the grocery store, although the chips I make with my homemade All Seasoning Spice are my favorite.

PREHEAT the oven to 375°F. Line a baking sheet with parchment paper or a silicone mat.

IN a small bowl, mix together the cheddar, mozzarella, and Parmesan until fully combined.

SPOON 1-tablespoon portions of the cheese mixture onto the baking sheet, making sure to leave 1 inch between them to allow room to spread while baking. Sprinkle the All Seasoning Spice over the cheese.

BAKE for 8 to 10 minutes, until just melted and bubbly. Start watching after 6 minutes to avoid burning. Let cool slightly and serve immediately. They are best when served warm out of the oven.

STORE the chips in a covered container in the refrigerator for up to 1 week.

NUTRITIONAL INFO (PER SERVING)
CALORIES 130, **FAT** 8.3g, **PROTEIN** 12.1g, **CARBS** 1.7g, **FIBER** 0.5g

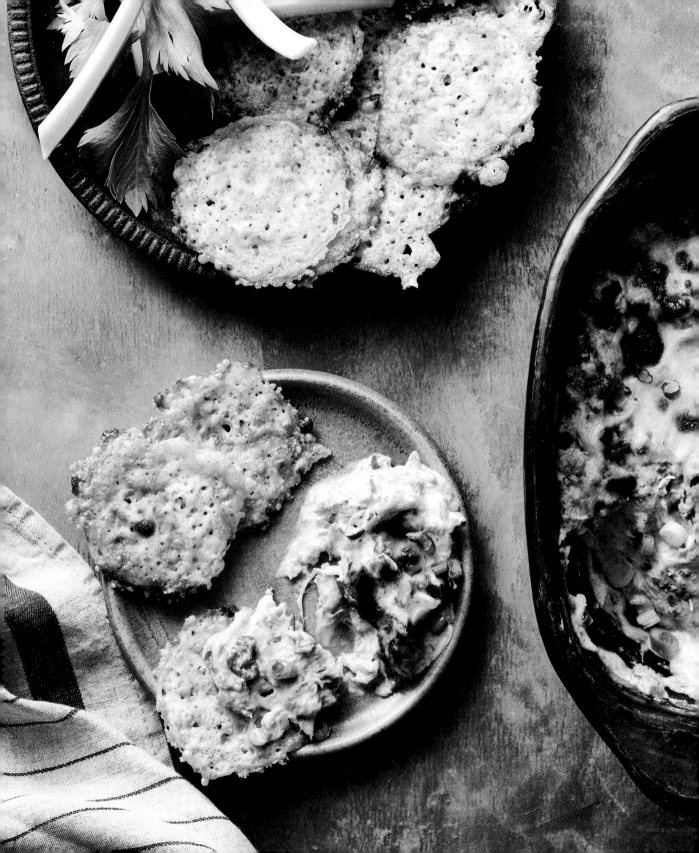

BACON CHEESEBURGER DIP

1 tablespoon extra-virgin olive oil

12 ounces 80 percent lean ground beef

4 ounces cream cheese, at room temperature

½ cup sour cream

1 tablespoon tomato paste

2 teaspoons yellow mustard

1 teaspoon ground cumin

1 teaspoon chili powder

½ teaspoon garlic powder

½ teaspoon onion powder

½ teaspoon black pepper

½ teaspoon ground cayenne pepper

3 dill pickles, diced

1 cup shredded cheddar cheese

5 slices Makin' Bacon (page 270), crumbled

Celery sticks, for dipping

MAKES 10 SERVINGS

This hearty dip recipe is a real party pleaser! Prepare it the night before and pop it in the oven to bake just before you're ready to serve. Add a bit more cayenne pepper or add fresh sliced jalapeños if you want it to be extra spicy.

PREHEAT the oven to 375°F. Spray a 9-inch square baking dish with cooking spray.

IN a large skillet over medium-high heat, heat the olive oil. Add the ground beef and cook, breaking it up with a spoon, until browned. Drain and discard the fat.

IN a medium bowl using a hand mixer, beat the cream cheese, sour cream, and tomato paste until smooth. Add the mustard, cumin, chili powder, garlic powder, onion powder, black pepper, and cayenne pepper and beat until smooth. Using a spoon, mix in the cooked ground beef, diced pickles, and ½ cup of shredded cheddar cheese.

TRANSFER the mixture to the prepared baking dish and top with the remaining ½ cup cheddar cheese and the crumbled bacon. Bake for 20 to 22 minutes, until the cheese is bubbly and golden brown. Serve with celery sticks, for dipping.

NUTRITIONAL INFO (PER SERVING)
CALORIES 233, **FAT** 18.1g, **PROTEIN** 14.1g, **CARBS** 3.5g, **FIBER** 0.6g

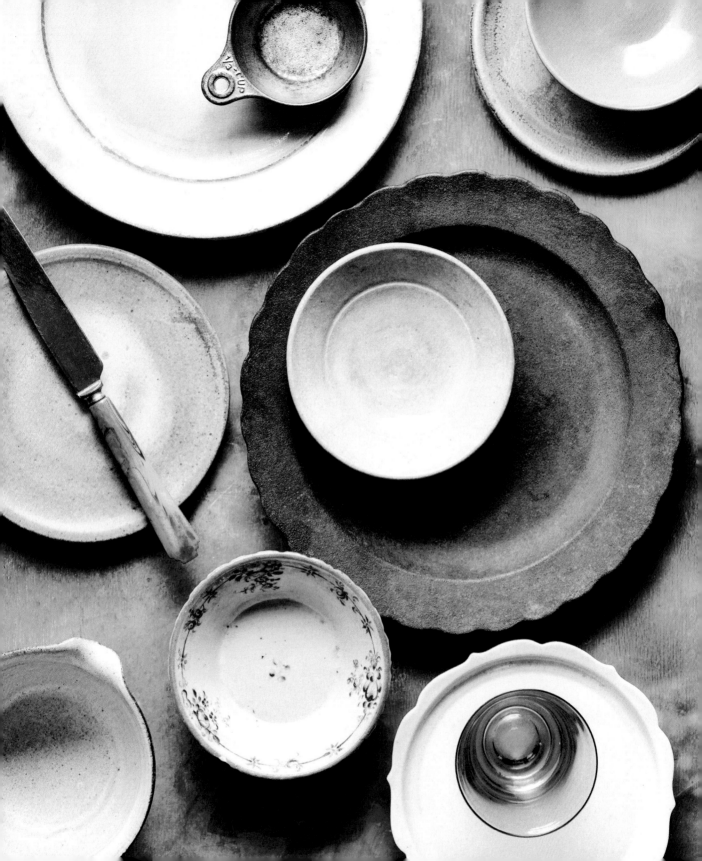

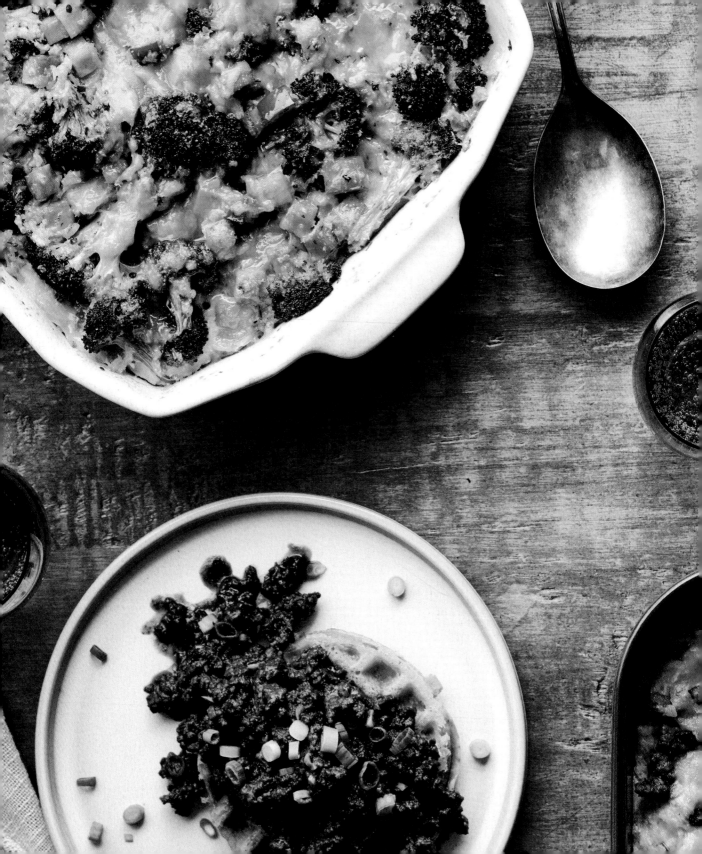

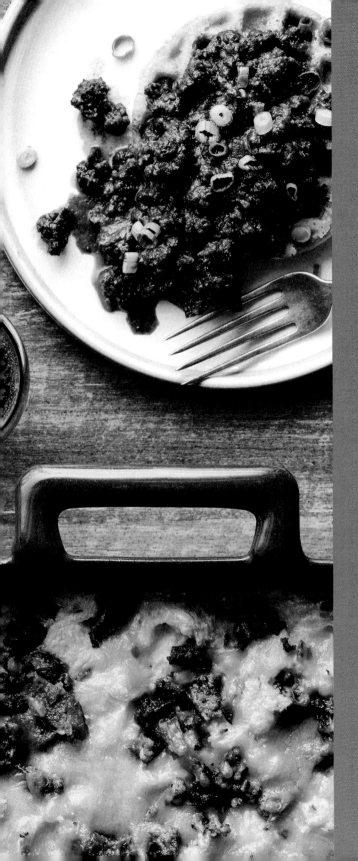

LUNCH & DINNER

CHILES RELLENOS CASSEROLE

2 (4-ounce) cans diced green chiles, drained

8 ounces shredded part-skim low-moisture mozzarella cheese

3 large eggs

1 (4-ounce) jar of sliced pimientos, drained

¾ cup heavy whipping cream

½ teaspoon salt

½ teaspoon black pepper

4 ounces shredded cheddar cheese

Chopped fresh cilantro, for garnish

Sour cream, for garnish

MAKES 6 SERVINGS

Instead of individually stuffing each chile with cheese, layer the ingredients in a baking dish and get all the flavor without all the work. What I really love about this recipe is that it makes a lot of leftovers, which will get you another meal, and it also doubles easily so it can feed a crowd.

PREHEAT the oven to 350°F. Spray an 8-inch square baking pan with cooking spray.

SPREAD the chiles over the bottom of the pan. In a large bowl, mix together the mozzarella, eggs, pimientos, cream, salt, and pepper and spread over the chiles. Top with the cheddar cheese.

BAKE for 35 minutes, or until the casserole is set and the cheese is golden brown. Garnish with cilantro and dollops of sour cream and serve hot.

NUTRITIONAL INFO (PER SERVING)
CALORIES 298, **FAT** 22.9g, **PROTEIN** 17.7g, **CARBS** 5.5g, **FIBER** 0.4g

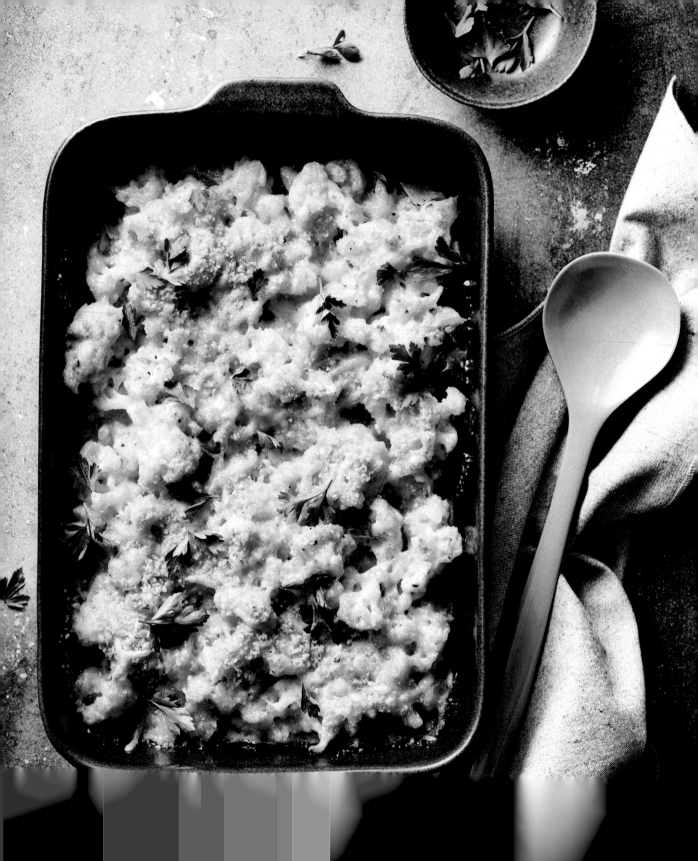

CAULI-MAC AND CHEESE BAKE

1 large head cauliflower, cut into florets

½ cup heavy whipping cream

2 ounces cream cheese, at room temperature

2 tablespoons unsalted butter

1 teaspoon dry mustard

1 teaspoon paprika

1 teaspoon salt

1 teaspoon black pepper

1 cup shredded sharp cheddar cheese

½ cup shredded Monterey Jack cheese

2 tablespoons chopped fresh parsley

MAKES 6 SERVINGS

Paprika adds a depth of flavor to this recipe that you will love. You can purchase frozen cauliflower to save time; just make sure you defrost it and drain the water before adding to the casserole. You could also add diced ham to make the casserole a complete, hearty meal.

BRING a large pot of water to a boil over high heat. Add the cauliflower and cook until tender, 5 to 7 minutes. Drain in a colander and set aside.

IN the same pot over medium heat, mix together the cream, cream cheese, butter, mustard, paprika, salt, and pepper and cook, stirring, until smooth. Add the cheddar and Monterey Jack cheese and stir until the cheese is melted and the mixture is smooth.

ADD the cauliflower and stir until completely coated in the sauce. Transfer to a large bowl, sprinkle with parsley, and serve.

NUTRITIONAL INFO (PER SERVING)
CALORIES 229, **FAT** 18.6g, **PROTEIN** 8.8g, **CARBS** 9g, **FIBER** 3.1g

GREEN BEAN CASSEROLE

1 cup sliced button
  mushrooms, optional

½ cup heavy whipping cream

4 ounces cream cheese, at
  room temperature

1 teaspoon prepared
  mustard

1 teaspoon Worcestershire
  sauce

½ teaspoon onion powder

½ teaspoon garlic powder

½ teaspoon xanthan gum or
  guar gum, if needed

1 (12- to 15-ounce) package
  frozen green beans

1 teaspoon salt

½ teaspoon black pepper

½ cup grated Parmesan
  cheese

½ cup pork panko or
  crushed pork rinds

MAKES 6 SERVINGS

My family always has this for Thanksgiving, but we love it so
much that we make it often throughout the year too. This is
one of the many recipes that calls for a cast-iron skillet. I swear,
there is something really special about cooking food in cast iron.
Everything tastes ten times better and the pan can go directly
from the stove into the oven. I'm lucky enough to have a big
assortment of cast-iron skillets that will probably last a lifetime,
and I use them all the time.

PREHEAT the oven to 350°F.

IN a large cast-iron pan over medium-high heat, mix together the
mushrooms, if using, cream, cream cheese, mustard, Worcestershire
sauce, onion powder, and garlic powder and cook until heated
through. If the sauce seems thin, add the xanthan gum. Add the
green beans and toss with the sauce. Season with salt and pepper
to taste.

BAKE for 20 minutes. Sprinkle the top with the Parmesan cheese
and pork panko and continue to bake for another 10 minutes, until
the casserole is bubbly and the cheese is browned. Serve hot.

NUTRITIONAL INFO (PER SERVING)
CALORIES 254, **FAT** 19g, **PROTEIN** 16.7g, **CARBS** 4.2g, **FIBER** 1g

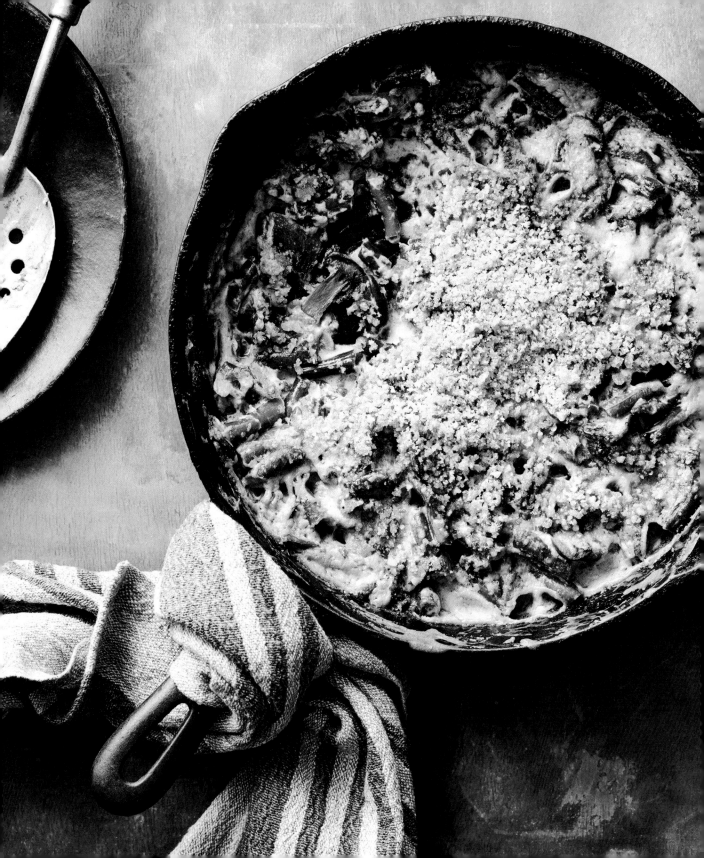

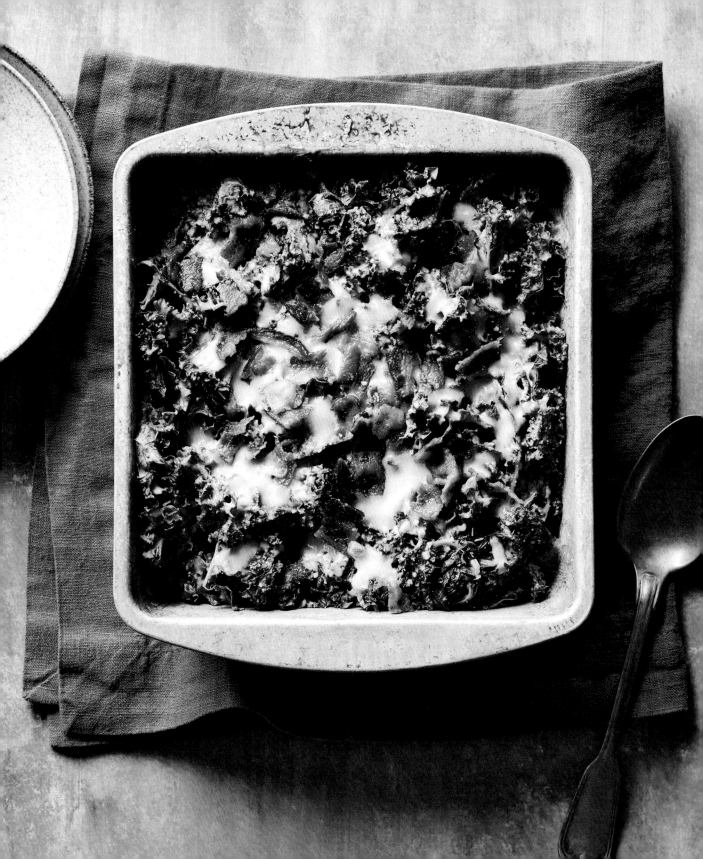

CREAMED KALE

3 cups chopped kale, stems removed

1 cup Basic Condensed Cream Soup (page 266)

1 teaspoon Italian seasoning

1 teaspoon salt

1 teaspoon black pepper

¼ cup shredded part-skim low-moisture mozzarella cheese

2 tablespoons grated Parmesan cheese

3 tablespoons crumbled Makin' Bacon (page 270)

MAKES 4 SERVINGS

Buy chopped kale in a microwave-safe bag at your local grocery store to save time. Just pop the bag in the microwave oven for 3 minutes and the work is already done for you.

PREHEAT the oven to 375°F. Have an 8-inch square baking dish ready.

IN a microwave-safe bowl, sprinkle the kale with 1 tablespoon water. Heat in the microwave oven for 3 minutes, or until the kale is tender. Spread the kale evenly in the baking dish.

POUR the condensed soup over the kale and sprinkle with the Italian seasoning, salt, and pepper. Sprinkle the cheeses and bacon over the top.

BAKE for 20 to 22 minutes, until the cheese is melted and lightly browned.

NUTRITIONAL INFO (PER SERVING)
CALORIES 409, **FAT** 24.2g, **PROTEIN** 11.1g, **CARBS** 2.8g, **FIBER** 0.4g

BROCCOLI BACON CASSEROLE

12 ounces broccoli florets, cut into 1-inch pieces

1 cup Basic Condensed Cream Soup (page 266)

1 teaspoon Italian seasoning

1 teaspoon salt

1 teaspoon black pepper

¾ cup shredded part-skim low-moisture mozzarella cheese

¼ cup grated Parmesan cheese

¼ cup crumbled Makin' Bacon (page 270)

MAKES 5 SERVINGS

Buy cut broccoli florets in a microwave-safe bag at your local grocery store to save time. Heat them in the microwave for 3½ minutes. No chopping needed.

PREHEAT the oven to 375°F. Have a 9-inch square baking dish ready.

IN a microwave-safe bowl, sprinkle the broccoli with 1 tablespoon water. Cook on high for 3½ minutes until the broccoli florets are tender. Transfer the broccoli to the baking dish.

POUR the condensed soup over the broccoli. Sprinkle with the Italian seasoning, salt, and pepper. Sprinkle the mozzarella, Parmesan, and bacon over the top.

BAKE for 20 to 22 minutes, until the cheese is melted and lightly browned. Serve hot.

NUTRITIONAL INFO (PER SERVING)
CALORIES 311, **FAT** 25.4g, **PROTEIN** 15.7g, **CARBS** 6.3g, **FIBER** 1.7g

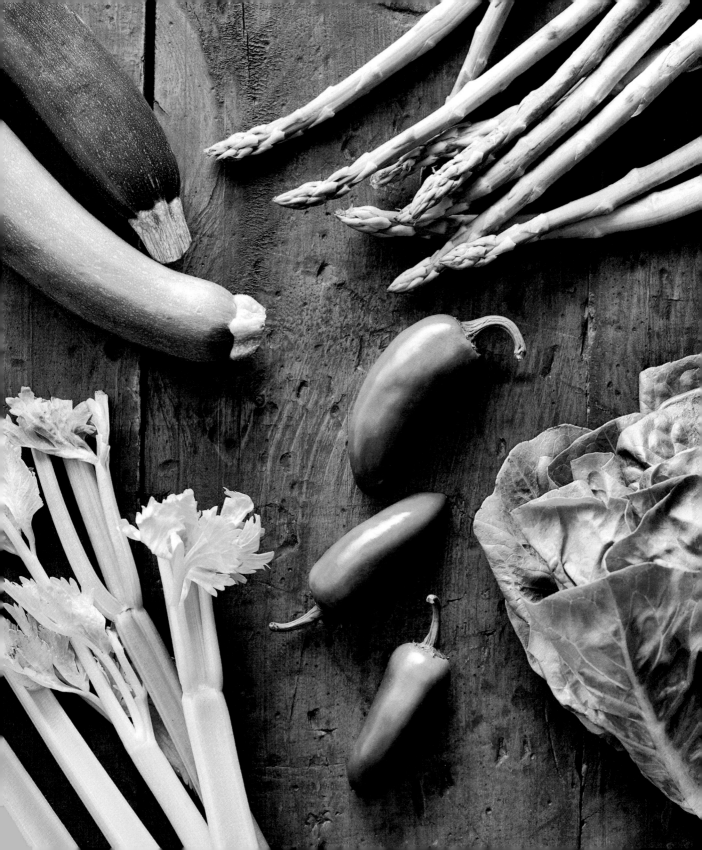

SALMON PATTIES

1 large egg

1 pound skinless salmon fillets, cut into ½-inch pieces

¼ cup blanched almond flour

¼ cup pork panko or crushed pork rinds

½ cup shredded part-skim low-moisture mozzarella cheese

2 tablespoons extra-virgin olive oil

2 tablespoons sliced green onions

1 tablespoon coconut aminos

1 tablespoon mayonnaise

1 teaspoon minced garlic

1 teaspoon salt

1 teaspoon black pepper

MAKES 9 PATTIES (9 SERVINGS)

If you are looking for a really simple and fast dinner idea, this is it. Serve the patties with a side salad and you'll have a balanced light lunch or dinner. You can buy pork panko in the bread section of most grocery stores, but if yours doesn't carry it, pulse pork rinds in a food processor.

PREHEAT the oven to 400°F. Line a baking sheet with parchment paper or a silicone mat.

IN a large bowl, whisk the egg. Add the salmon, almond flour, pork panko, mozzarella, olive oil, green onions, coconut aminos, mayonnaise, garlic, salt, and pepper and mix until combined.

DIVIDE the mixture into nine equal patties. Place the patties on the prepared baking sheet and bake for 18 to 20 minutes, until golden brown. Serve warm.

NUTRITIONAL INFO (PER SERVING)
CALORIES 196, **FAT** 11g, **PROTEIN** 20.8g, **CARBS** 1.3g, **FIBER** 0.2g

TUNA CASSEROLE

1 (12-ounce) can tuna in oil, drained

1½ cups shredded Colby Jack cheese

3 ounces cream cheese, at room temperature

⅓ cup sour cream

1 jalapeño pepper, diced

2 tablespoons diced onion

1 tablespoon chopped fresh parsley

2 teaspoons Old Bay seasoning

2 (7-ounce) bags shirataki fettuccine noodles, drained

½ cup pork panko or crushed pork rinds

MAKES 5 SERVINGS

This recipe is a keto twist on an old-time favorite my family used to make. To reduce the carb count, instead of regular noodles I use shirataki noodles, which are made with a type of yam. Once I discovered them, a world of options for keto cuisine opened up.

PREHEAT the oven to 350°F. Have a 7- by 11-inch baking dish ready.

IN a medium bowl, mix together the tuna, 1 cup of the Colby Jack cheese, the cream cheese, sour cream, jalapeño, onion, parsley, and Old Bay until fully combined.

RINSE the shirataki noodles under cold water for about 3 minutes.

IN a medium skillet over medium heat, cook the shirataki noodles to get as much moisture out of them as possible, about 5 minutes, flipping the noodles halfway through to dry both sides. Add the noodles to the tuna mixture and mix until fully combined.

TRANSFER the noodle mixture to the baking dish and top with the remaining ½ cup Colby Jack and the pork panko. Bake for 30 minutes, or until heated through. Serve hot.

NUTRITIONAL INFO (PER SERVING)
CALORIES 422, **FAT** 29.4g, **PROTEIN** 33.5g, **CARBS** 5g, **FIBER** 0.9g

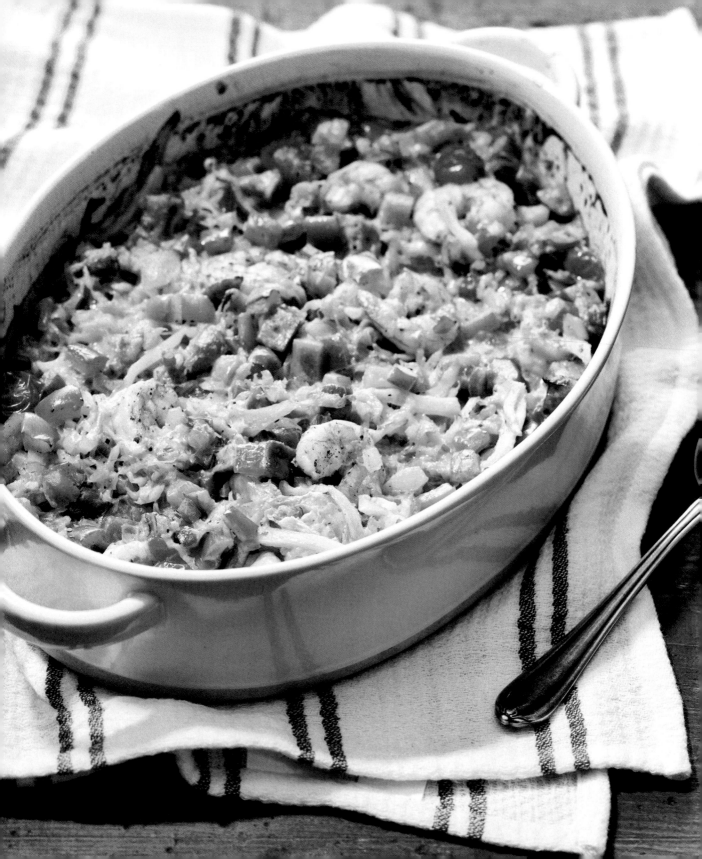

CREAMY CAJUN SHRIMP CASSEROLE

1 tablespoon extra-virgin olive oil

1 red bell pepper, diced

1 green bell pepper, diced

¼ cup diced onion

1 (10-ounce) bag angel hair coleslaw

½ cup chopped cherry tomatoes

1 tablespoon butter

1 cup heavy whipping cream

½ cup grated Parmesan cheese

2 teaspoons Cajun seasoning

1 teaspoon black pepper

12 ounces cooked small shrimp, peeled

2 cups diced kielbasa sausage

MAKES 6 SERVINGS

This casserole has a mild flavor so if you really like heat, add a pinch of cayenne pepper for some extra spice. Cajun seasoning, which can be purchased at your local supermarket, is a blend of salt, garlic, paprika, black pepper, onion powder, and cayenne pepper. This recipe makes a meal when you serve it with cauli-mashed potatoes, cauli-rice, or a side salad.

PREHEAT the oven to 350°F. Have a 9- by 13-inch baking dish ready.

IN a medium skillet over medium heat, heat the olive oil. Add the red and green pepper and onion and cook, stirring, until the onion is translucent. Add the coleslaw and cherry tomatoes and cook, stirring, until the coleslaw is tender, about 5 minutes.

IN a small saucepan over medium heat, melt the butter. Add the cream and bring to a simmer. Add the Parmesan cheese, Cajun seasoning, and black pepper and cook, stirring, until the sauce begins to thicken.

PLACE the coleslaw mixture, shrimp, and kielbasa in the baking dish. Pour the cream mixture over the top and mix until well combined. Bake for 30 minutes, or until heated through. Serve hot.

NUTRITIONAL INFO (PER SERVING)
CALORIES 245, **FAT** 17g, **PROTEIN** 17.8g, **CARBS** 6.4g, **FIBER** 1.7g

CHICKEN, HAM, AND CHEESE CASSEROLE

8 boneless, skinless chicken thighs

1 teaspoon Italian seasoning

1 teaspoon salt

1 teaspoon black pepper

1½ cups Basic Condensed Cream Soup (page 266)

8 slices deli ham

8 slices Swiss cheese

1 cup shredded part-skim low-moisture mozzarella cheese

MAKES 8 SERVINGS

The classic chicken cordon bleu recipe is a time-consuming dish that requires you to pound chicken until it's thin and then roll it up around ham and cheese. But here, I've simply layered the ingredients so you get the same flavors with a lot less time and effort. Bring it to a potluck—everyone will love it.

PREHEAT the oven to 350°F.

PLACE the chicken thighs in a 15- by 10-inch baking dish and sprinkle with the Italian seasoning, salt, and pepper. Bake for 22 minutes.

DRIZZLE the chicken with condensed soup, then place a slice of ham and a slice of Swiss cheese over each chicken thigh. Sprinkle the mozzarella over the top. Bake for an additional 10 minutes, or until the chicken reaches an internal temperature of 165°F and the cheese is melted and golden brown. Serve hot.

NUTRITIONAL INFO (PER SERVING)
CALORIES 441, **FAT** 23.2g, **PROTEIN** 53.3g, **CARBS** 2g, **FIBER** 0.1g

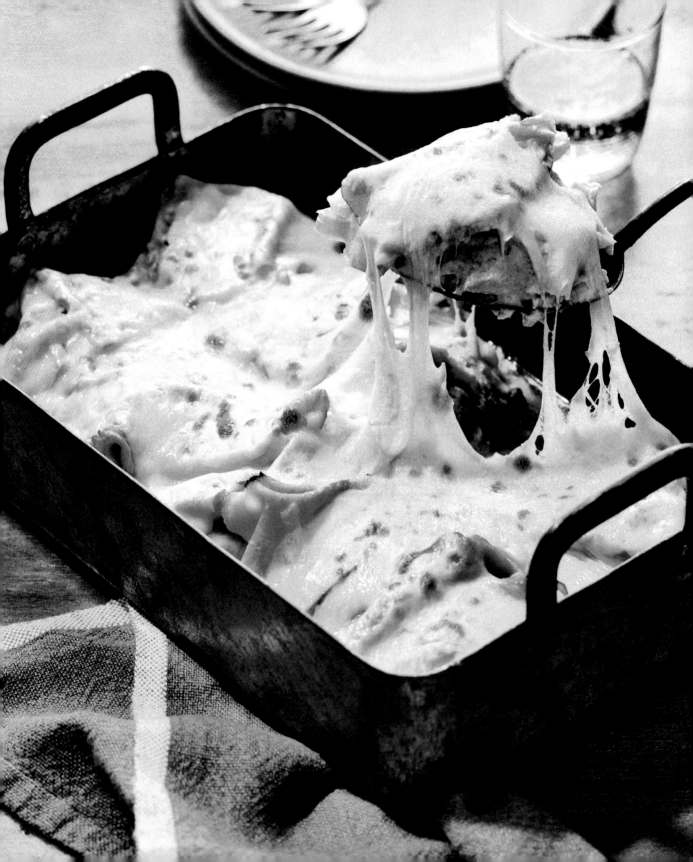

CHICKEN, BACON, AND BRUSSELS SPROUTS CASSEROLE

12 ounces Brussels sprouts, cut in half

3 tablespoons extra-virgin olive oil

1 teaspoon salt

6 strips sugar-free nitrite-free bacon, diced

2½ cups diced or shredded cooked chicken

1 cup shredded Gruyère cheese

½ cup cherry tomatoes, chopped

⅓ cup sour cream

¼ cup ricotta cheese

2 ounces cream cheese, at room temperature

1 tablespoon Worcestershire sauce

1 teaspoon All Seasoning Spice (page 274)

1 teaspoon onion powder

MAKES 6 SERVINGS

If you think you don't like Brussels sprouts, think again. Roasting them brings out their sweetness and gives this dish a wonderful sweet-savory flavor that you'll want to eat again and again.

PREHEAT the oven to 425°F. Line a baking sheet with parchment paper or a silicone mat. Have a 9- by 13-inch baking dish ready.

IN a medium bowl, mix together the Brussels sprouts, olive oil, and salt. Arrange the Brussels sprouts and bacon on the prepared baking sheet. Bake for 20 minutes, until they are caramelized. Set aside.

LOWER the oven temperature to 350°F.

IN a medium bowl, mix together the chicken, Gruyère, tomatoes, sour cream, ricotta, cream cheese, Worcestershire sauce, All Seasoning Spice, and onion powder. Add the Brussels sprouts and bacon, mix until combined, and transfer to the baking dish. Bake for 30 minutes, or until heated through.

NUTRITIONAL INFO (PER SERVING)
CALORIES 485, **FAT** 34.3g, **PROTEIN** 36g, **CARBS** 8.6g, **FIBER** 2.4g

CREAMY CHICKEN AND GREEN BEAN CASSEROLE

3 ounces cream cheese, at room temperature

½ cup sour cream

6 slices Makin' Bacon (page 270), crumbled

½ tablespoon All Seasoning Spice (page 274)

2 cups shredded cooked chicken

12 ounces fresh green beans

½ cup shredded cheddar cheese

½ cup pork panko or crushed pork rinds

MAKES 4 SERVINGS

We've added a good amount of healthy fats and bacon to make the casserole rich and flavorful. Double the recipe and you'll have enough to feed a large family.

PREHEAT the oven to 350°F. Have an 11- by 7-inch baking dish ready.

IN a medium bowl, mix together the cream cheese, sour cream, bacon, and All Seasoning Spice. Add the chicken and stir to combine.

IN a microwave-safe bowl, combine the green beans with ¼ cup water and heat in the microwave oven for 3 to 5 minutes, until tender. Add the green beans to the chicken mixture and transfer to the baking dish. Sprinkle the cheddar cheese and pork panko over the top.

BAKE for 30 minutes, or until the casserole is bubbly and the cheese is melted and golden brown. Serve immediately.

NUTRITIONAL INFO (PER SERVING)
CALORIES 548, **FAT** 36.5g, **PROTEIN** 45.5g, **CARBS** 8.1g, **FIBER** 1.8g

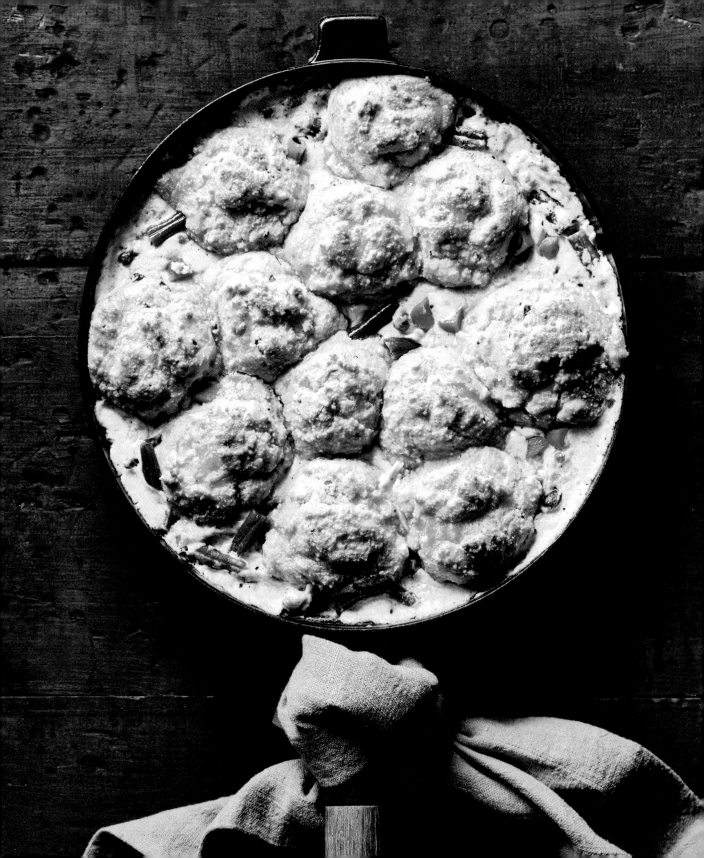

CHEESY BISCUIT–CHICKEN POT PIE

FILLING

⅓ cup butter

1 cup frozen mixed vegetables

⅓ cup chopped onion

1 teaspoon minced garlic

½ teaspoon salt

¼ teaspoon black pepper

¼ teaspoon poultry seasoning

¾ cup Stovetop Chicken Stock (page 264) or store-bought

3 ounces cream cheese

1 cup heavy whipping cream

2 teaspoons Frank's RedHot hot sauce

1 teaspoon xanthan gum

2½ cups cooked shredded chicken

CHEESY BISCUITS

1½ cups blanched almond flour

1 tablespoon baking powder

½ teaspoon garlic powder

½ teaspoon onion powder

¼ teaspoon salt

2 large eggs

½ cup sour cream

4 tablespoons butter, melted

½ cup shredded cheddar cheese

Chopped fresh parsley, optional

MAKES 10 SERVINGS

I took an all-time favorite classic recipe—pot pie—and made it keto friendly. This might be the perfect keto comfort food. Even your non-keto friends will be impressed. I've used my popular biscuit recipe and used it as a topping, and I think it's a winner!

PREHEAT the oven to 450°F.

FOR THE FILLING

IN a large cast-iron skillet, melt the butter over medium heat. Add the mixed vegetables, onion, garlic, salt, pepper, and poultry seasoning. Cook, stirring, until the vegetables are tender, 7 to 10 minutes. Set aside.

IN a separate skillet over medium heat, mix together the stock, cream cheese, cream, and hot sauce and cook, stirring, until the cheese is melted and the mixture is smooth. Sprinkle in the xanthan gum and stir until the sauce thickens.

ADD the cooked chicken and the cream mixture to the cooked vegetables in the cast-iron skillet and stir to combine. Set aside.

FOR THE CHEESY BISCUITS

IN a medium bowl, mix together the almond flour, baking powder, garlic powder, onion powder, and salt. Add the eggs, sour cream, melted butter, and cheddar cheese and mix until the mixture comes together into a stiff dough.

USING a tablespoon, drop equal portions of the dough over the vegetable mixture. Bake for about 30 to 35 minutes, until a toothpick inserted into the centers of the biscuits comes out clean. Sprinkle with the parsley, if you like, and serve hot.

NUTRITIONAL INFO (PER SERVING)
CALORIES 414, **FAT** 27.6g, **PROTEIN** 20.8g, **CARBS** 9.2g, **FIBER** 1.6g

EASY CHICKEN FLORENTINE

4 slices sugar-free nitrite-free bacon

4 boneless, skinless chicken breasts

1 teaspoon salt

½ teaspoon black pepper

1 tablespoon extra-virgin olive oil

8 ounces button mushrooms, sliced

1 small onion, chopped

1 tablespoon minced garlic

1 (10-ounce) bag fresh spinach

1 recipe Basic Condensed Cream Soup (page 266)

1 cup grated Parmesan cheese

¼ cup heavy whipping cream

1 tablespoon fresh lemon juice

1 tablespoon Italian seasoning

2 cups shredded part-skim low-moisture mozzarella cheese

MAKES 8 SERVINGS

Chicken can get boring if you eat it a lot, like we do in our family. So I'm always trying to jazz it up in new ways. The traditional chicken Florentine originated in Florence and features fresh spinach. We love this keto version and I'm sure you will too. For an extra hearty dinner, serve over shirataki angel hair noodles or cauli-mashed potatoes.

PREHEAT the oven to 350°F. Have ready a 9- by 13-inch baking dish. Line a plate with paper towels.

IN a large skillet over medium heat, cook the bacon until crisp, about 8 minutes. Remove the bacon with a slotted spoon and let drain on the paper towel–lined plate. Reserve the bacon grease in the skillet.

SEASON the chicken with the salt and pepper. Add the chicken to the skillet and cook over medium heat until browned, about 3 minutes on each side. They don't need to be cooked through. Transfer the chicken to a plate and set aside.

ADD the olive oil, mushrooms, onions, and garlic to the skillet and cook, stirring, until the onion is translucent, about 5 minutes. Add the spinach, toss with the mushrooms, and cook, stirring, until the spinach is wilted but not cooked all the way through, about 3 minutes. Transfer the mixture to the baking dish and arrange the chicken breasts on top.

IN the same skillet, mix together ¼ cup water, the condensed soup, Parmesan cheese, cream, lemon juice, and Italian seasoning. Pour the mixture over the chicken breasts, making sure to cover each one. Place the bacon over the chicken breasts and sprinkle 1 cup of the mozzarella cheese over the top.

(continued)

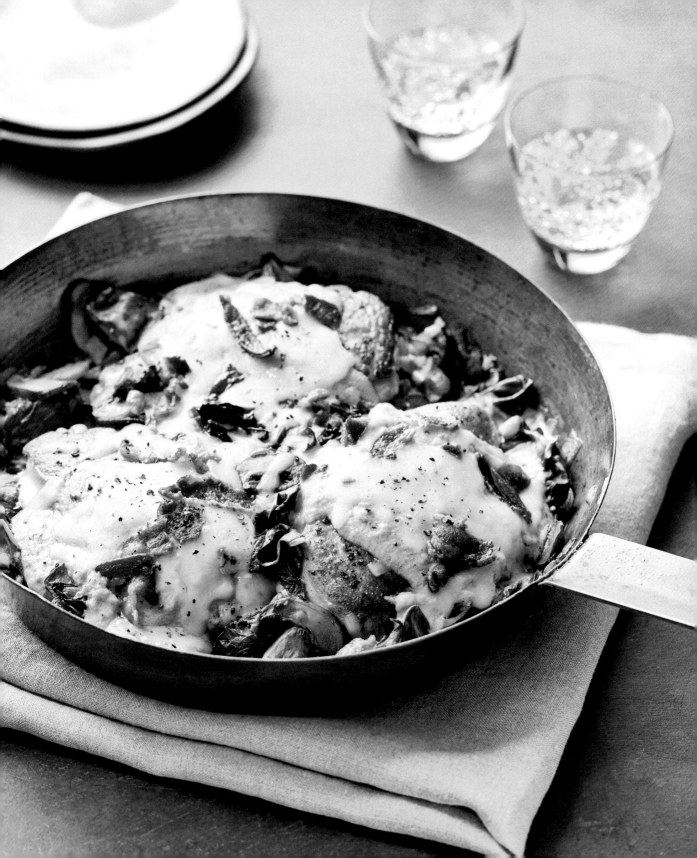

Cover with aluminum foil and bake for 30 to 40 minutes, until the chicken is fully cooked and reaches an internal temperature of 165°F.

REMOVE the foil, sprinkle the remaining 1 cup mozzarella over the top, and bake, uncovered, for another 5 to 10 minutes, until the cheese is golden brown. Serve immediately.

NUTRITIONAL INFO (PER SERVING)
CALORIES 342, **FAT** 25.1g, **PROTEIN** 23.8g, **CARBS** 5.7g, **FIBER** 0.6g

SALSA VERDE CHICKEN CASSEROLE

1 (16-ounce) bag frozen cauliflower florets

1½ cups salsa verde

1 cup sour cream

8 ounces cream cheese, at room temperature

¼ cup minced fresh cilantro

½ teaspoon minced garlic

2 cups shredded Mexican cheese blend or Monterey Jack cheese

2 cups shredded cooked chicken

1 (10-ounce) can Ro*Tel mild diced tomatoes and green chilies, drained, optional

MAKES 8 SERVINGS

This recipe uses a wonderful green salsa made with tomatillos to turn boring chicken into a meal that everyone will enjoy. Salsa verde is easy to find at most grocery stores. While you are there, buy a rotisserie chicken if you don't have cooked chicken at home. This is the perfect dinner idea for those super-busy days when you don't have any time to think about making dinner.

PREHEAT the oven to 350°F. Have a 9- by 13-inch baking dish ready.

PLACE the cauliflower in a microwave safe bowl and heat in the microwave oven for about 5 minutes, until tender.

IN a medium bowl, combine the cauliflower, salsa verde, sour cream, cream cheese, cilantro, garlic, and 1 cup of the Mexican cheese blend. Add the shredded chicken and the Ro*Tel, if using, and mix until combined. Spread the mixture evenly in the baking dish. Sprinkle the remaining 1 cup cheese over the top.

BAKE for 30 minutes, or until the casserole is heated through and the cheese is golden brown. Serve hot.

NUTRITIONAL INFO (PER SERVING)
CALORIES 373, **FAT** 26.7g, **PROTEIN** 24.8g, **CARBS** 8.2g, **FIBER** 1.1g

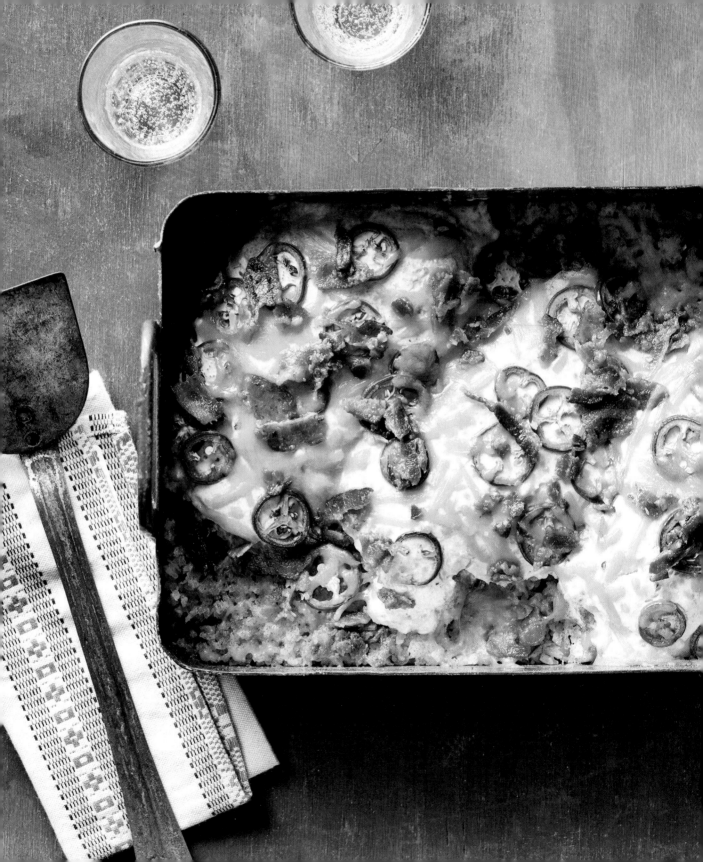

CHICKEN–JALAPEÑO POPPER CASSEROLE

8 ounces cream cheese, at room temperature

⅓ cup mayonnaise

⅓ cup grated Parmesan cheese

1 teaspoon prepared mustard

1 teaspoon sriracha or Frank's RedHot hot sauce

1 (10-ounce) bag frozen cauliflower rice, thawed

4 boneless, skinless chicken breasts

½ teaspoon onion powder

½ teaspoon garlic powder

½ teaspoon paprika

2 to 4 jalapeños peppers (fresh or pickled), sliced

½ cup shredded cheddar cheese

6 strips Makin' Bacon (page 270), crumbled

MAKES 8 SERVINGS

Here's a super-easy recipe for you—all you need to do is layer the ingredients and bake. The juices from the chicken soak into the riced cauliflower while baking which makes this taste so good! Make it more spicy by using fresh jalapeños and their seeds, or go milder by removing the seeds. My family doesn't like meals really spicy so I go one step further and use pickled jalapeños, which are even milder.

PREHEAT the oven to 350°F. Have a 9- by 13-inch baking dish ready.

IN a medium bowl, mix together the cream cheese, mayonnaise, Parmesan cheese, mustard, and sriracha. Set aside.

SPREAD the cauliflower rice evenly in the baking dish. Arrange the chicken breasts on the cauliflower and sprinkle with onion powder, garlic powder, and paprika. Spread the cream cheese mixture on top of each chicken breast, covering them completely. Top with the sliced jalapeños, cheddar cheese, and bacon.

BAKE for 35 to 40 minutes, until the chicken is fully cooked and reaches an internal temperature of 165°F. Serve hot.

NUTRITIONAL INFO (PER SERVING)
CALORIES 326, **FAT** 29.2g, **PROTEIN** 11.4g, **CARBS** 4.9g, **FIBER** 1g

CHICKEN AND CHEESE ENCHILADAS

3 boneless, skinless chicken breasts

5 ounces cream cheese

1 (4.5-ounce) can diced green chiles

1 teaspoon salt

1 teaspoon black pepper

½ teaspoon ground cumin

½ teaspoon chili powder

½ teaspoon garlic powder

4 medium zucchini, thinly sliced into long ribbons

1 (20-ounce) can Rosarita enchilada sauce

1½ cups shredded Monterey Jack cheese

1 cup crumbled queso fresco

½ cup sour cream, for serving

MAKES 4 SERVINGS

This recipe uses zucchini in place of regular pasta noodles. To cut them, simply slice zucchini lengthwise into thin strips (about ⅛ inch thick) using a mandoline or sharp knife. When all of the flavors bake together, it will be hard to even notice you used zucchini instead of regular noodles.

PREHEAT the oven to 375°F. Have a 9- by 13-inch baking dish ready.

IN a large saucepan, place the chicken in a single layer. Pour enough water over the chicken to cover by about 1 inch. Bring the water to a boil over medium-high heat. Lower the heat to medium-low, cover, and simmer until the chicken is fully cooked and reaches an internal temperature of 165°F. Drain, let cool, and shred the chicken using two forks.

IN a bowl, mix together the shredded chicken, cream cheese, green chiles, salt, pepper, cumin, chili powder, and garlic powder until thoroughly combined.

LAY 5 or 6 zucchini slices on a clean work surface, overlapping the edges to create a large rectangle. Place about ¼ cup of the chicken mixture across one short end and roll up the zucchini. Repeat to make about 8 rolls. The first one or two will be a little messy but you'll get the hang of it. Transfer the zucchini rolls to the baking dish. Top with the enchilada sauce, Monterey Jack cheese, and queso fresco.

BAKE for about 45 minutes, until bubbling and the cheese is golden brown. Top with dollops of sour cream and serve hot.

NUTRITIONAL INFO (PER SERVING)
CALORIES 159, **FAT** 13g, **PROTEIN** 8.6g, **CARBS** 8.6g, **FIBER** 1.6g

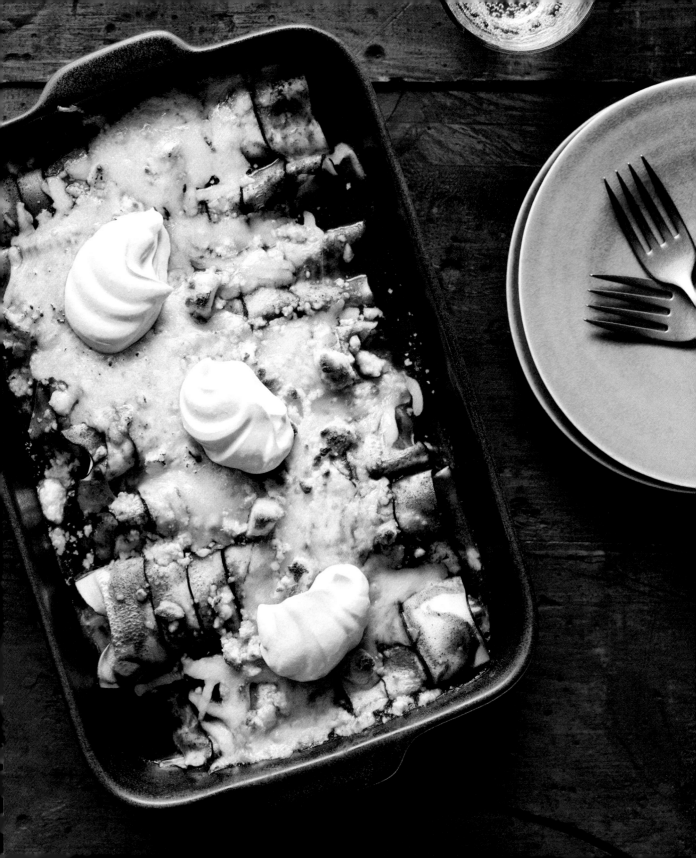

BRINED TURKEY

1 cup kosher salt

4 to 6 garlic cloves, peeled

3 bay leaves

2 sprigs fresh rosemary, leaves removed and roughly chopped

2 sprigs fresh thyme

1 tablespoon Montreal Steak seasoning

1 tablespoon black peppercorns

1 (12-pound) turkey, thawed

MAKES 12 SERVINGS

After looking for a way to give my turkey the best flavor with a tender and juicy outcome, I finally figured out how to make my bird come out perfect every time. It's all about the brining, which is a chemical process that breaks down the meat proteins and makes the most tender turkey you'll ever taste. And something wonderful happens when you mix salt and spices that help the turkey retain all its juices so it's always moist and never dry. You may never want to make your turkey any other way. Honestly, it's the best. Don't forget to give the turkey plenty of time to thaw, which will take a minimum of 3 days in the refrigerator. I use a turkey steam bag when I roast my turkey but it's not required.

IN a large pot over medium-high heat, mix together the salt, garlic, bay leaves, rosemary, thyme, steak seasoning, peppercorns, and 1 gallon water and bring to a boil to create a brine. Set aside to cool.

PLACE the turkey into a large poultry bag or a clean cooler (like I do) and pour in the brine. If using a poultry bag, seal the bag and place the turkey in the refrigerator. If using a cooler, place a bag of ice over the turkey and cover with the lid. You should brine for 1 hour for each pound of meat. For example, a 12-pound turkey should be brined for 12 hours. Be sure to keep the turkey refrigerated the entire time or add ice to the cooler as needed to keep it cold.

PREHEAT the oven to 350°F. Place the turkey in a roasting pan and roast for 13 minutes for each pound of the turkey (or 15 minutes for each pound of a stuffed turkey). For example, a 12-pound unstuffed turkey should roast for just over 2½ hours. The internal temperature of the turkey (taken at the thickest part) should read 165°F.

NUTRITIONAL INFO (PER SERVING)
CALORIES 509, **FAT** 12.3g, **PROTEIN** 92.5g, **CARBS** 0.9g, **FIBER** 0.3g

PAN-GRILLED STEAK WITH SHRIMP AND BACON BUTTER

3 (8-ounce) rib eye steaks

2 teaspoons garlic powder

1 teaspoon paprika

1 teaspoon salt

1 teaspoon black pepper

1 pound raw shrimp, peeled and deveined

1 teaspoon All Seasoning Spice (page 274)

4 slices sugar-free nitrite-free bacon

8 tablespoons butter, at room temperature

2 teaspoons minced garlic cloves

2 teaspoons minced fresh thyme

MAKES 3 SERVINGS

Let me tell you about bacon butter. Combining bacon, garlic, thyme, and butter makes the best topping for steak you will ever have. Add shrimp to the recipe and you'll wonder why you never made this before now. To cook the steaks, I've used a reverse sear method in which the steak is baked first and then seared. So good.

PREHEAT the oven to 250°F. Place a baking rack in a large baking pan. Line a plate with paper towels.

SEASON the steaks with the garlic powder, paprika, salt, and black pepper. Place the steaks on the rack in the pan and bake for 25 minutes.

IN a large bowl, season the shrimp with the All Seasoning Spice and let sit for 25 minutes.

IN a skillet over medium heat, cook the bacon until crispy, 3 to 4 minutes on each side. Remove the bacon and reserve the bacon grease in the skillet. Cool the bacon on the paper towel–lined plate, then crumble.

IN a medium bowl using a hand mixer, beat 4 tablespoons of the butter until creamy. Add the bacon, garlic, and 1 teaspoon of the thyme and mix with a spoon until combined. Cover the bowl with plastic wrap and refrigerate.

IN the skillet with the reserved bacon grease, melt the remaining 4 tablespoons butter over medium-high heat and add the remaining 1 teaspoon thyme. Add the steaks and sear for 3 to 5 minutes per side, spooning the butter mixture over the steak occasionally. Transfer the steaks to a plate and let rest.

(continued)

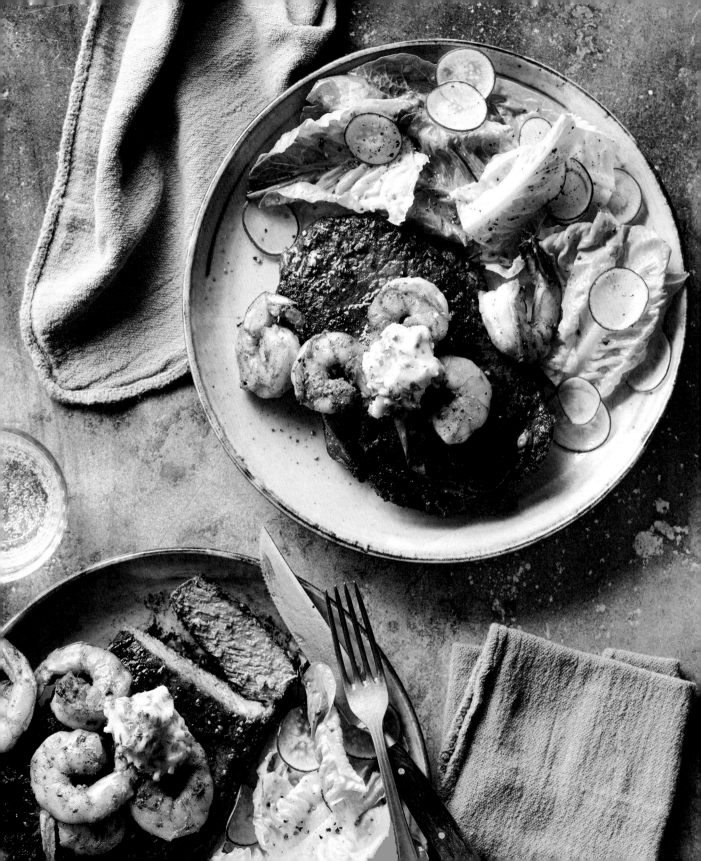

TO the same skillet over medium heat, add the shrimp and cook for 2 minutes. Turn the shrimp and continue to cook, stirring, until pink, another 2 to 3 minutes.

TO serve, place each steak on a plate, top with the shrimp, and dollop with the bacon butter.

NUTRITIONAL INFO (PER SERVING)
CALORIES 615, **FAT** 48.8g, **PROTEIN** 42.2g, **CARBS** 3.8g, **FIBER** 0.8g

SALISBURY STEAK WITH LOW-CARB GRAVY

SALISBURY STEAK

2 pounds 90 percent lean ground beef

1 cup pork panko or crushed pork rinds

1 large egg

1 tablespoon dried parsley

2 teaspoons Worcestershire sauce

1 teaspoon salt

1 teaspoon black pepper

½ teaspoon garlic powder

1 tablespoon extra-virgin olive oil

3 tablespoons butter

1 onion, thinly sliced

8 ounces button mushrooms, sliced

3 sprigs fresh thyme

GRAVY

2 cups Pressure Cooker Bone Broth (page 265) or store-bought bone broth

½ cup heavy whipping cream

4 tablespoons butter

1 teaspoon black pepper

½ teaspoon xanthan gum

2 sprigs fresh thyme

MAKES 6 SERVINGS

While my husband has joined me on this keto lifestyle journey, what keeps him here is recipes like this one. He can't tell the difference between a traditional Salisbury steak and my low-carb version. It's worth doubling or even tripling this recipe and freezing the excess so you can serve it to your family any time.

PREHEAT the oven to 350°F. Have a 9- by 13-inch baking dish ready.

FOR THE SALISBURY STEAKS

IN a large bowl, mix together the ground beef, pork panko, egg, parsley, Worcestershire, salt, pepper, and garlic powder until well combined. Using your hands, form the mixture into six patties.

IN a large skillet over medium-high heat, heat the olive oil. Add the patties and cook until browned on both sides. Transfer to the baking dish and set aside.

IN the same skillet over medium-high heat, melt the butter. Add the onion, mushrooms, and thyme and cook, stirring, until the onions have softened, 2 to 3 minutes. Spoon the onion mixture over the patties.

FOR THE GRAVY

IN the same skillet over medium-high heat, mix together the bone broth, cream, butter, pepper, xanthan gum, and thyme and bring to a boil. Lower the heat to low and cook, whisking occasionally, until the gravy reduces and reaches your desired level of thickness, 10 to 15 minutes.

POUR the gravy over the steaks and cover the pan with aluminum foil. Bake for 35 to 40 minutes, until the centers of steak patties are cooked through.

NUTRITIONAL INFO (PER SERVING)
CALORIES 583, **FAT** 34.5g, **PROTEIN** 60.4g, **CARBS** 5.7g, **FIBER** 1.4g

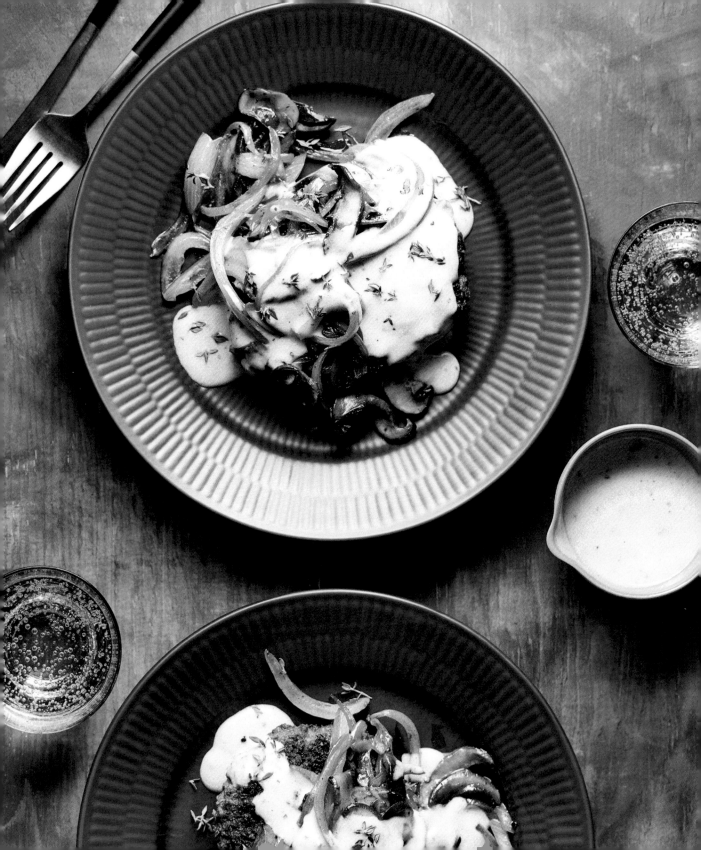

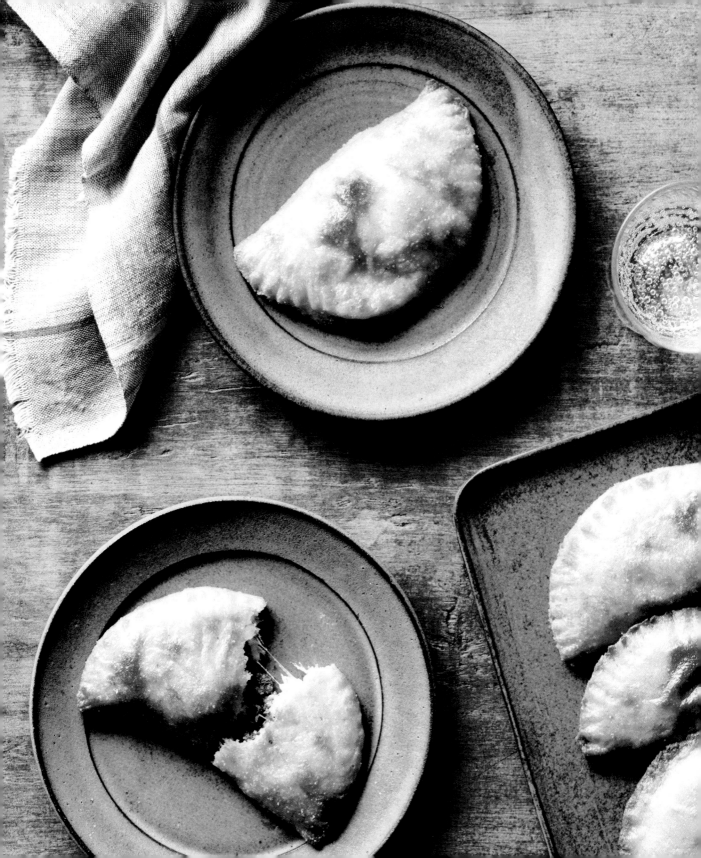

CHEESY BEEF EMPANADAS

FILLING

1 tablespoon extra-virgin olive oil

1 pound 90 percent lean ground beef

2 garlic cloves, minced

1 jalapeño pepper, diced

2 teaspoons tomato paste

1 teaspoon unsweetened cocoa powder

1 teaspoon onion powder

1 teaspoon dried oregano

1 teaspoon ground cumin

1 teaspoon chili powder

1 teaspoon salt

½ teaspoon black pepper

½ teaspoon paprika

DOUGH

2 cups shredded part-skim low-moisture mozzarella cheese

2 ounces cream cheese, at room temperature

1 cup blanched almond flour

½ cup shredded Monterey Jack or pepper Jack cheese

1 large egg

MAKES 10 MEDIUM-SIZE EMPANADAS (10 SERVINGS)

If you are missing savory pastry, this recipe will hit the spot. The empanadas are great to make ahead and warm up in the microwave. Like most keto doughs, this one is easier to work with when it's warm. Don't be afraid to reheat it in the microwave and then continue with the recipe.

FOR THE FILLING

IN a medium skillet over medium-high heat, heat the oil. Add the ground beef and cook, breaking it up with a wooden spoon, until cooked through. Drain and discard the fat. Add the garlic, jalapeño, tomato paste, cocoa powder, onion powder, oregano, cumin, chili powder, salt, black pepper, and paprika and mix well. Set aside to cool.

FOR THE DOUGH

PREHEAT the oven to 350°F. Line a baking sheet with parchment paper or a silicone mat. Have two large sheets of parchment paper ready.

IN a microwave-safe bowl, mix together the mozzarella cheese and cream cheese and heat in the microwave oven for 1 to 1½ minutes, until the cheese has melted. Add the almond flour and mix together until all the ingredients come together. Knead the dough until smooth, then divide into two pieces. If the dough becomes hard to knead, heat it in the microwave oven for 20 to 30 seconds and continue kneading.

PLACE one piece of dough on a sheet of parchment paper and cover with the other sheet of parchment. Using a rolling pin, roll the dough to ¼ inch thick. Using a 4-inch round cookie cutter, cut out 5 rounds of dough. Repeat with the remaining piece of dough; you should have 10 rounds in total.

(continued)

PLACE about 2 tablespoons of the filling in the center of a dough circle and top it with 1 tablespoon of shredded Jack cheese. Fold the dough over to cover the filling and fold the ends inwards to seal the empanada. Repeat with the rest of the filling, cheese, and dough. Place the empanadas on the prepared baking sheet.

IN a small bowl, whisk the egg with 1 tablespoon water until frothy to make an egg wash. Brush the empanadas with the egg wash. Bake for 12 to 15 minutes, until the empanadas are golden brown.

NUTRITIONAL INFO (PER SERVING)
CALORIES 208, **FAT** 10.2g, **PROTEIN** 16.2g, **CARBS** 4.8g, **FIBER** 0.8g

TACO CASSEROLE

1 tablespoon extra-virgin
   olive oil

1 small onion, diced

2 pounds 90 percent lean
   ground beef

1 teaspoon salt

1 teaspoon black pepper

½ teaspoon xanthan gum,
   optional

¼ cup Taco Seasoning
   (page 275)

1 (15-ounce) can black
   soybeans, drained

1½ cups shredded Mexican
   cheese blend

1 (10-ounce) can Ro*Tel mild
   diced tomatoes and green
   chilies

1 (4-ounce) can diced green
   chiles

4 large eggs

¼ cup heavy whipping cream

Black olives, optional

OPTIONAL TOPPINGS

Chopped fresh cilantro,
   chopped green onions, sour
   cream, shredded lettuce,
   sriracha, sliced jalapeño
   peppers, sliced avocado

MAKES 8 SERVINGS

Mexican food often calls for beans, which are not on the keto diet, but I have found that black soybeans are a great substitute. They are higher in some phytonutrients, including antioxidants, which is another reason I like them so much. Look for them in natural food stores, but if you have trouble finding them (like I do), you can get them online.

PREHEAT the oven to 350°F. Have a 9- by 11-inch baking pan ready.

IN a large skillet over medium heat, heat the oil. Add the onion and cook, stirring, until translucent, 4 to 5 minutes. Add the ground beef, salt, and pepper and cook, breaking up the beef with a wooden spoon, until browned. Add the xanthan gum, if using, to thicken up the liquid. Add the taco seasoning and mix thoroughly. Add the soy beans, 1 cup of the shredded cheese, Ro*Tel, and green chiles and stir until well combined. Transfer the mixture to the baking pan.

IN a small bowl, mix together the eggs and cream. Pour the egg mixture into the beef mixture in the casserole dish and stir until fully combined. Sprinkle with the remaining ½ cup cheese and black olives, if using.

BAKE for 35 to 40 minutes, until the casserole is bubbly and the cheese is golden brown. Serve with individual bowls of the optional toppings on the side.

NUTRITIONAL INFO (PER SERVING)
CALORIES 737, **FAT** 64.2g, **PROTEIN** 34.3g, **CARBS** 6.1g, **FIBER** 1.6g

JALAPEÑO POPPER–STUFFED MEAT LOAF

1½ pounds ground beef or ground pork (or a mixture of both)

¼ cup chopped onion

½ teaspoon minced garlic

½ cup pork panko, crushed pork rinds, ground flaxseed, or blanched almond flour

2 large eggs

1 tablespoon Italian seasoning

1 tablespoon dry mustard

1 teaspoon coconut aminos or soy sauce

½ teaspoon black pepper

8 ounces cream cheese, at room temperature

2 jalapeño peppers, diced

½ cup crumbled Makin' Bacon (page 270)

5 tablespoons AlternaSweets low-carb classic tomato ketchup

MAKES 8 SERVINGS

This recipe evolved when I noticed how my family loved the Chicken–Jalapeño Popper Casserole (page 97)—so I figured out how to make a meat loaf version with similar flavors. I used pork panko here, but if you use flavored varieties of pork rinds, like salt and vinegar or barbecue you'll change how it tastes. Crush them with your hands or give them a few pulses in a food processor to make crumbs.

PREHEAT the oven to 400°F. Spray a loaf pan with cooking spray.

IN a large bowl, mix together the ground beef, onion, garlic, pork panko, eggs, Italian seasoning, mustard, liquid aminos, and pepper. (I often use my hands to mix it all together, just like my grandma.)

TRANSFER half the meat mixture to the prepared loaf pan and press evenly into the pan. Spread the softened cream cheese over the meat mixture. Scatter the jalapeños and crumbled bacon over the cream cheese. Press the remaining meat mixture into the pan. Spread the ketchup over the top of the meat loaf. Cover the pan with aluminum foil and bake for 1 hour, until the meat loaf is cooked through.

WRAP any leftovers tightly in aluminum foil and refrigerate for 4 days, or freeze for up to 1 month.

NUTRITIONAL INFO (PER SERVING)
CALORIES 291, **FAT** 15.7g, **PROTEIN** 23.5g, **CARBS** 8.4g, **FIBER** 0.6g

VARIATION

MINI MEAT LOAVES: If you want to get dinner on the table a little sooner, layer the meat mixture and other ingredients into two smaller loaf pans and bake for only 30 to 40 minutes. I've done this when my family was hungry and wanted dinner pronto.

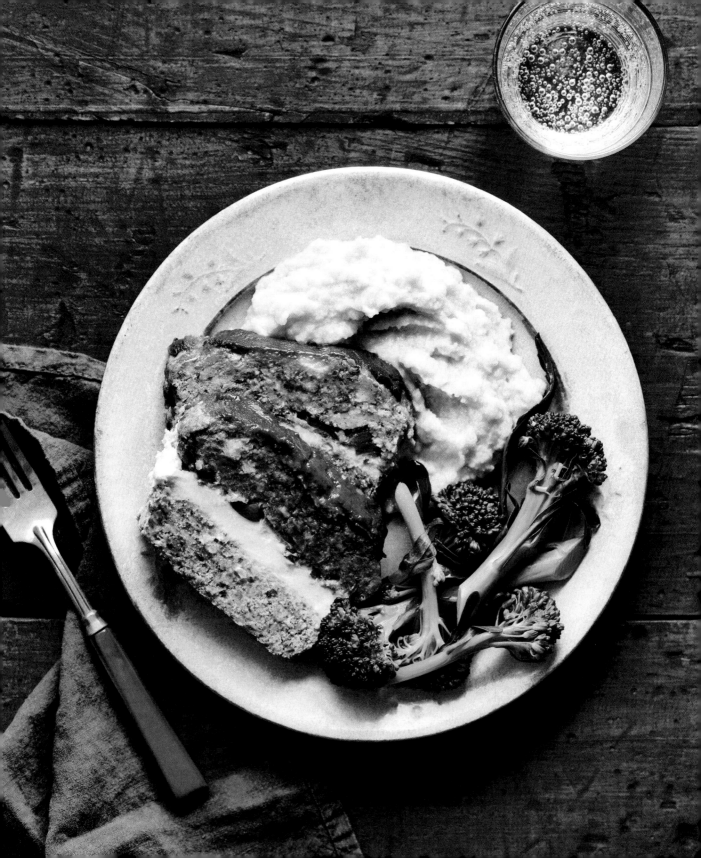

SAUSAGE HASH CASSEROLE

10 ounces green cabbage, thinly sliced, or 1 (10-ounce) package angel hair coleslaw

1 green bell pepper, diced

1 red bell pepper, diced

½ cup diced onion

¼ cup extra-virgin olive oil

1 tablespoon All Seasoning Spice (page 274)

1 (12-ounce) package kielbasa sausage, cut into diagonal ½-inch-thick pieces

MAKES 6 SERVINGS

This recipe is perfect when you want a lighter dinner that's loaded with vegetables. You can cut up a green cabbage, or save time by purchasing angel hair coleslaw at your local grocery store.

PREHEAT the oven to 350°F.

IN a 9-inch square baking pan, spread out the cabbage evenly. Add the green and red bell peppers and onion. Drizzle with the olive oil and mix slightly until the vegetables are covered. Sprinkle with the All Seasoning Spice and top with the kielbasa.

COVER the pan with aluminum foil and bake for 20 minutes, until the cabbage is completely soft and the sausage is cooked through.

NUTRITIONAL INFO (PER SERVING)
CALORIES 239, **FAT** 19.4g, **PROTEIN** 8.6g, **CARBS** 9.3g, **FIBER** 2.4g

MEATBALL CASSEROLE

1 pound 90 percent lean ground beef

1 pound spicy pork sausage meat

2 cups shredded part-skim low-moisture mozzarella cheese

1/2 cup pork panko or crushed pork rinds

1/3 cup grated Parmesan cheese

2 large eggs

2 teaspoons onion powder

2 teaspoons minced garlic

1/2 teaspoon Italian seasoning

2 cups Rao's marinara sauce

1 cup shredded cheddar cheese

1/2 cup chopped fresh basil

MAKES 8 SERVINGS

This low-carb meal is absolutely fabulous in every way imaginable. It's a clear winner with my whole family. And you really can't mess it up. A mix of ground beef and spicy pork sausage makes the meatballs very flavorful, and crushed pork rinds fill in for the more traditional bread crumbs. Serve with a side salad.

PREHEAT the oven to 400°F. Spray a 9- by 13-inch baking dish with cooking spray.

IN a large bowl, mix together the ground beef, sausage, 1 cup of the mozzarella, the pork panko, Parmesan, eggs, onion powder, garlic, and Italian seasoning until combined. I usually mix it with my (clean) hands. Roll the mixture into 1-inch meatballs and transfer to the baking dish.

BAKE for 15 to 20 minutes, until cooked through. Drain any excess oil from the baking dish. Top the meatballs with the marinara, remaining 1 cup mozzarella, and the cheddar cheese and bake for an additional 5 to 10 minutes, until the cheese is melted. Garnish with the basil.

NUTRITIONAL INFO (PER SERVING)
CALORIES 554, **FAT** 35.9g, **PROTEIN** 46.6g, **CARBS** 8.8g, **FIBER** 1.3g

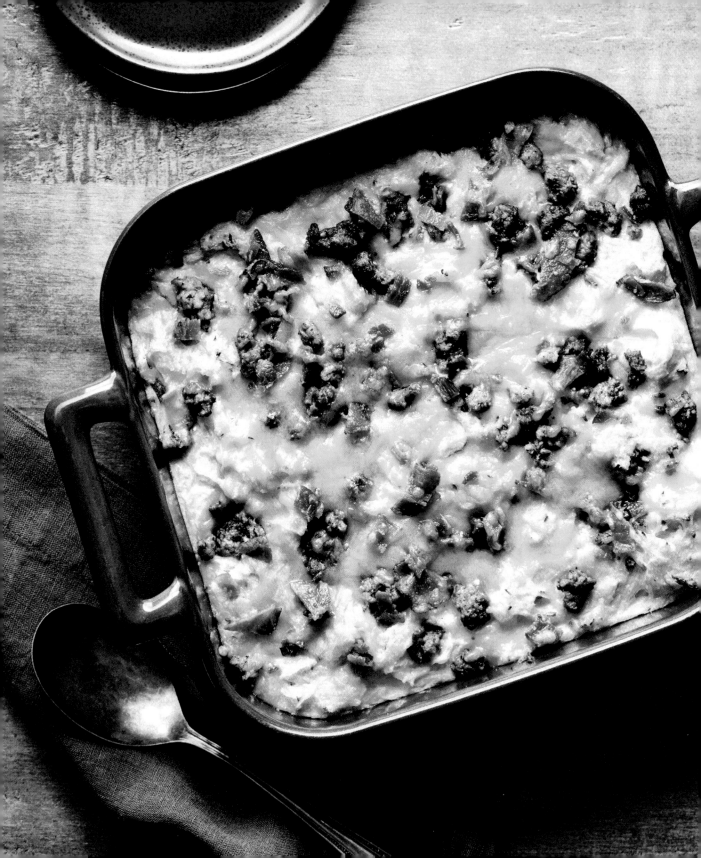

MILLION DOLLAR SPAGHETTI SQUASH CASSEROLE

1 large spaghetti squash

1 tablespoon extra-virgin olive oil

½ pound ground beef

½ pound ground pork

3 large eggs

⅓ cup heavy whipping cream

2 cups shredded cheddar cheese

½ cup grated Romano cheese

½ cup ricotta cheese

1 tablespoon chopped fresh parsley

1 tablespoon sriracha

1 teaspoon Worcestershire sauce

2 teaspoons salt

1 teaspoon black pepper

1 teaspoon garlic powder

1 teaspoon onion powder

1 teaspoon dry mustard

½ cup crumbled Makin' Bacon (page 270)

MAKES 6 SERVINGS

This recipe can be made in a flash when you bake the spaghetti squash in a pressure cooker. It comes out perfectly tender every single time.

PREHEAT the oven to 350°F. Have a 9- by 13-inch baking dish ready.

CUT the squash in half, remove the seeds, and add to an Instant Pot. Add ½ cup water and seal with the lid. Press the manual setting and set it to high pressure for 10 minutes. When the cycle ends, perform a quick release. Use a fork to shred the squash out of the shell and set aside.

IN a large skillet over medium-high heat, heat the oil. Add the ground beef and ground pork and cook, breaking up the meat with a wooden spoon, until browned. Remove from the heat.

IN a medium bowl, whisk the eggs with the cream. Add 1 cup of the cheddar cheese, the Romano cheese, ricotta, parsley, sriracha, Worcestershire, salt, pepper, garlic powder, onion powder, and dry mustard and mix until fully combined. Add the spaghetti squash and browned meat and mix until fully combined.

POUR the mixture into the baking dish and top with the remaining 1 cup cheddar cheese and the bacon. Bake for 30 minutes, until the casserole is bubbly and the cheese is golden brown.

NUTRITIONAL INFO (PER SERVING)
CALORIES 330, **FAT** 23.1g, **PROTEIN** 23.5g, **CARBS** 7.1g, **FIBER** 1g

CHEESEBURGER PIE

6 thick-cut slices sugar-free nitrite-free bacon

½ cup diced onion

½ pound 80 percent lean ground beef

½ pound ground pork

½ cup diced dill pickles, plus more for topping

¼ cup beef broth

2 tablespoons tomato paste

2 teaspoons dry mustard

1 teaspoon minced garlic

1 teaspoon salt

½ teaspoon black pepper

½ teaspoon dried thyme

½ teaspoon dried sage

½ cup shredded cheddar cheese

1 prebaked Savory Pie Shell (page 244)

Shredded lettuce, for topping

Diced tomato, for topping

MAKES 1 (8-INCH) PIE (8 SERVINGS)

This is my husband's favorite recipe and he requests it often. It's a fun twist on the usual cheeseburger flavor. The hearty meal is best served with a side of your favorite vegetables or a salad. I like to make the pie crust ahead of time and freeze it so I'll always have one ready to go when I want to make this recipe.

PREHEAT the oven to 350°F. Line a plate with paper towels.

IN a large skillet over medium heat, cook the bacon until slightly crispy, then transfer to the paper towel–lined plate to cool. Reserve the bacon grease in the skillet. Cut the bacon into small pieces and set aside.

IN the same skillet over medium-high heat, heat the bacon grease. Add the onion and cook, stirring, until translucent, 4 to 5 minutes. Add the ground beef and pork and cook, breaking the meat up with a wooden spoon, until no longer pink. Drain any excess oil. Add the pickles, broth, tomato paste, dry mustard, garlic, salt, pepper, thyme, and sage and stir to combine. Add the bacon and continue to cook, stirring, until fully combined and thickened.

SPRINKLE 1 tablespoon of the cheddar cheese over the bottom of the pie shell, add the beef mixture, and top with the remaining cheddar. Bake for 10 to 12 minutes, until the edges of the pie crust are golden brown and the cheese has fully melted. Top with lettuce, diced tomato, and additional chopped pickles.

NUTRITIONAL INFO (PER SERVING)
CALORIES 220, **FAT** 14.1g, **PROTEIN** 19.5g, **CARBS** 3.2g, **FIBER** 0.5g

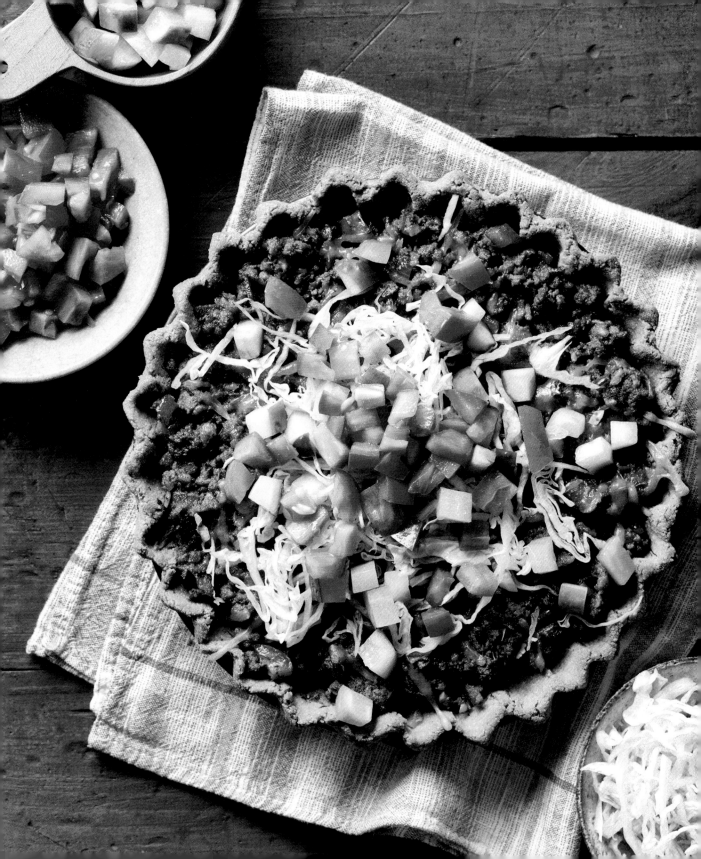

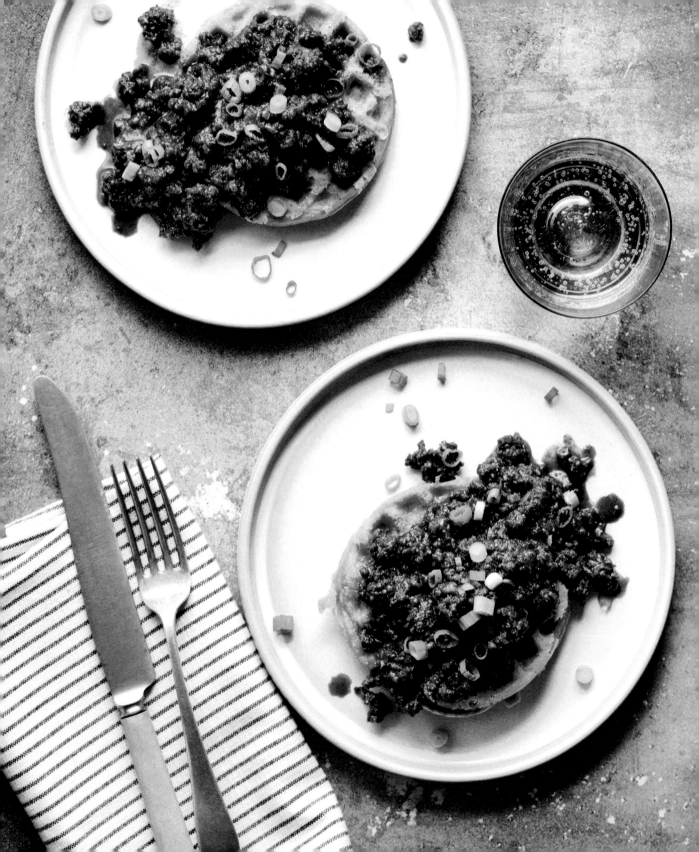

SLOPPY JOE CHAFFLES

SLOPPY JOE TOPPING

1 tablespoon extra-virgin olive oil

1 pound ground beef

½ cup Pressure Cooker Bone Broth (page 265) or store-bought

3 tablespoons tomato paste

1 tablespoon chili powder

1 teaspoon onion powder

1 teaspoon minced garlic

1 teaspoon coconut aminos or soy sauce

1 teaspoon cocoa powder, optional

1 teaspoon Swerve brown sugar sweetener

1 teaspoon dry mustard

½ teaspoon paprika

½ teaspoon salt

¼ teaspoon pepper

CORNBREAD CHAFFLE

2 large eggs

1 cup shredded cheddar cheese

10 slices jalapeño pepper, diced very small (pickled or fresh)

2 teaspoons Frank's RedHot hot sauce

½ teaspoon corn extract, optional

Pinch salt

Sliced green onion, optional

SERVES 4

The cocoa is optional in this recipe, but I highly recommend using it because it intensifies the flavors of the sloppy joe topping. If you use the corn extract, the chaffles will taste like real cornbread!

FOR THE SLOPPY JOE TOPPING

IN a large skillet over medium-high heat, heat the oil. Add the ground beef and cook, breaking it up with a wooden spoon, until browned. Add the bone broth, tomato paste, chili powder, onion powder, garlic, coconut aminos, cocoa, sweetener, dry mustard, paprika, salt, and pepper and stir to combine. Bring to a simmer and continue to cook, stirring occasionally until thickened and heated through, while you make the chaffles.

FOR THE CHAFFLES

PREHEAT a mini waffle maker according to the manufacturer's instructions.

IN a small bowl, whisk the eggs. Add the cheddar cheese, jalapeños, hot sauce, corn extract, if using, and the salt.

SPRAY the waffle maker with nonstick cooking spray. Pour one-fourth of the batter into the waffle maker and cook for about 4 minutes, or until golden brown. Repeat with the remaining batter to make four chaffles. For a crispier crust, add 1 teaspoon shredded cheese to the waffle maker and let cook for 30 seconds before adding the batter.

PLACE the chaffles on plates, pour the warm sloppy joe mixture over the tops, top with green onions, if using, and serve.

NUTRITIONAL INFO (PER SERVING)
CALORIES 156, **FAT** 3.9g, **PROTEIN** 25.8g, **CARBS** 3.9g, **FIBER** 1.2g

BLT CHAFFLE SANDWICH

1 large egg

½ cup shredded part-skim low-moisture mozzarella

1 tablespoon diced green onion

½ teaspoon Italian seasoning

1 tablespoon mayonnaise

Lettuce

5 slices Makin' Bacon (page 270)

Sliced tomato

MAKES 1 SANDWICH (2 SERVINGS)

No more breadless sandwiches when a chaffle can take the place of bread.

PREHEAT a mini waffle maker according to the manufacturer's instructions.

IN a small bowl, whisk the egg. Add the mozzarella, green onion, and Italian seasoning and mix until well combined.

POUR half of the batter into the waffle maker and cook for 4 minutes, or until golden brown. Repeat with the remaining batter. For a crispier crust, add 1 teaspoon shredded cheese to the waffle maker and let cook for 30 seconds before adding the batter.

SPREAD each chaffle with ½ tablespoon mayonnaise. Layer one chaffle with lettuce, bacon, and tomato and top with the second chaffle. Cut in half and serve.

NUTRITIONAL INFO (PER HALF SANDWICH)
CALORIES 183, **FAT** 13.9g, **PROTEIN** 10.8g, **CARBS** 3.6g, **FIBER** 0.6g

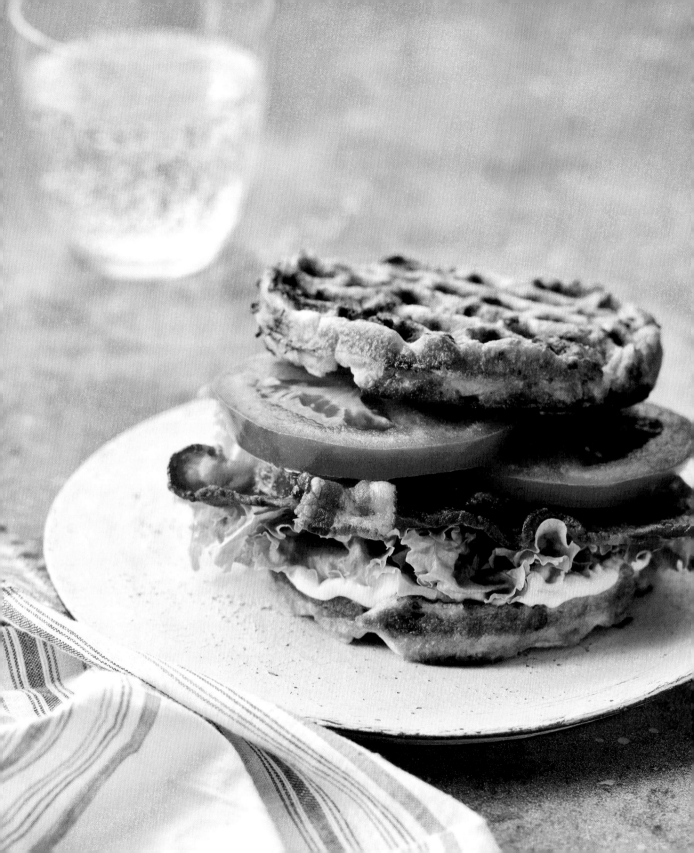

STUFFING CASSEROLE

8 ounces pork sausage meat

3 large eggs

8 tablespoons butter, melted

⅓ cup sour cream

2 cups blanched almond flour

2 teaspoons baking powder

3 tablespoons dried parsley

1 teaspoon dried sage

1 teaspoon dried rosemary

1 teaspoon salt

½ teaspoon garlic powder

½ teaspoon onion powder

½ cup shredded cheddar cheese

1 tablespoon extra-virgin olive oil

1 small onion, diced

1 cup sliced button mushrooms

1 cup diced celery

1 cup Stovetop Chicken Stock (page 264)

MAKES 12 SERVINGS

Stuff the Brined Turkey (page 100) with this stuffing for your holiday dinner, or serve it as a casserole on the side.

PREHEAT the oven to 350°F. Grease a 10- by 12-inch baking dish.

IN a medium skillet over medium heat, cook the sausage, breaking it up with a wooden spoon, until browned. Transfer half of the sausage to a bowl and set aside to cool. Leave the remaining sausage in the skillet.

IN a medium bowl using a hand mixer, beat the eggs until slightly frothy. Add 4 tablespoons of the butter and the sour cream and beat on medium speed until smooth. Add the sausage from the bowl, the almond flour, baking powder, parsley, sage, rosemary, salt, garlic powder, and onion powder and mix until fully combined. Fold in the cheddar cheese.

SPREAD the mixture in the baking dish and bake for 25 to 30 minutes, until golden brown and a toothpick inserted into the center comes out clean. Transfer the pan to a wire rack, cut the stuffing into 1-inch squares, and let cool in the pan.

ADD the olive oil to the skillet with the sausage and set over medium heat. Add the remaining 4 tablespoons butter, the onion, mushrooms, and celery and cook, stirring, until the vegetables are tender, about 10 minutes. Add the stock and stir to combine.

POUR the mixture into the baking dish and gently mix until well combined. Bake for 10 minutes, or until hot throughout and slightly browned on top.

NUTRITIONAL INFO (PER SERVING)
CALORIES 296, **FAT** 20g, **PROTEIN** 10.1g, **CARBS** 6.4g, **FIBER** 1.1g

COWBOY PORK CASSEROLE

½ pound pork sausage meat

1 (12-ounce) package riced cauliflower

2 cups shredded Colby Jack cheese

8 ounces cream cheese, at room temperature

1 cup sour cream

3 tablespoons dried parsley

2 tablespoons chili powder

1 tablespoon dried dill

1 tablespoon onion powder

1 tablespoon garlic powder

2 teaspoons salt

1 teaspoon black pepper

1 teaspoon smoked paprika

½ teaspoon dried oregano

1 pound (about 2 cups) shredded Pulled Pork (page 271)

MAKES 12 SERVINGS

I like to make the pulled pork recipe on the weekend so it will be ready to go during the week. But if you are tight on time, purchase pre-cooked pulled pork from your local grocery store.

PREHEAT the oven to 350°F. Have a 9- by 13-inch baking pan ready.

IN a large skillet over medium heat, cook the sausage, breaking it up with a wooden spoon, until no longer pink, 5 to 7 minutes. Add the cauliflower rice and cook, stirring, for about 5 minutes.

IN a large bowl, mix together 1 cup of the Colby Jack, the cream cheese, sour cream, parsley, chili powder, dill, onion powder, garlic powder, salt, pepper, paprika, and oregano until well combined. Add the pulled pork and sausage and cauliflower mixture and stir until fully combined.

POUR the mixture into the baking dish and sprinkle with the remaining 1 cup Colby Jack. Bake for 40 minutes, or until the casserole is bubbly and the cheese is golden brown. Serve hot.

NUTRITIONAL INFO (PER SERVING)
CALORIES 285, **FAT** 21.6g, **PROTEIN** 14.3g, **CARBS** 10.5g, **FIBER** 3g

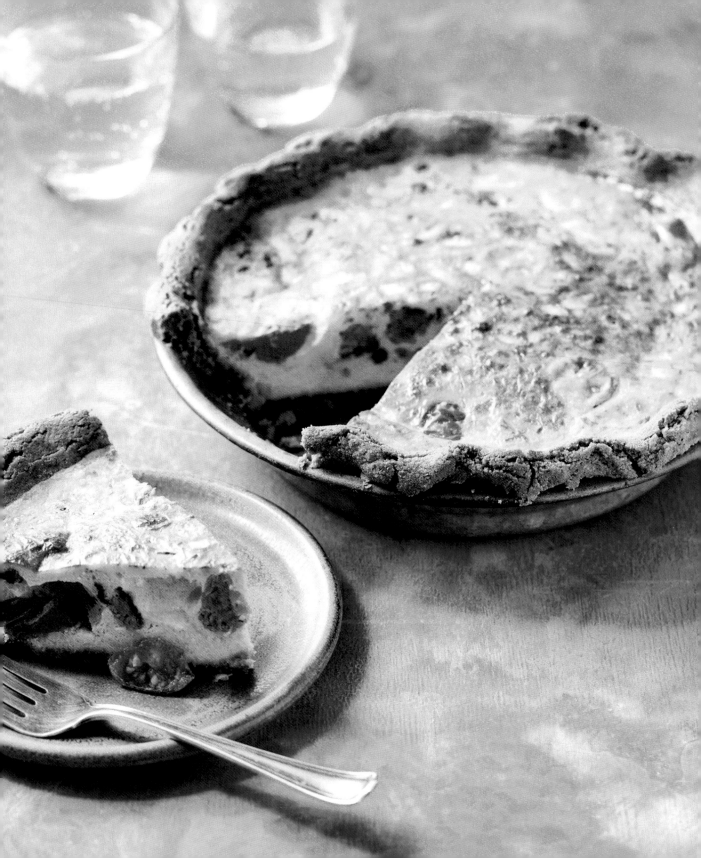

SAUSAGE QUICHE

½ pound pork sausage meat

6 large eggs

1 cup shredded Romano cheese

⅓ cup sour cream

1 tablespoon sriracha

½ teaspoon garlic powder

½ teaspoon onion powder

½ teaspoon dried thyme

½ teaspoon salt

½ teaspoon black pepper

½ cup chopped cherry tomatoes

1 unbaked Savory Pie Shell (page 244)

MAKES 1 (8-INCH) PIE (10 SERVINGS)

This is a great recipe to make ahead of time. It's very hearty and will keep you full for hours, and of course it's delicious. The savory crust is absolutely delightful.

PREHEAT the oven to 350°F.

IN a medium skillet over medium heat, cook the sausage, breaking it up with a wooden spoon, until no longer pink, about 5 minutes. Drain and discard the fat.

IN a medium bowl, whisk the eggs until frothy. Add the Romano cheese, sour cream, sriracha, garlic powder, onion powder, thyme, salt, pepper, and cherry tomatoes and mix together until fully combined. Add the sausage and mix to combine.

POUR the egg mixture into the pie shell. Fit 2-inch-wide strips of aluminum foil around the pie shell edge to prevent it from burning.

BAKE for 40 to 45 minutes, until fully cooked and a toothpick inserted in the center comes out clean. Serve hot.

NUTRITIONAL INFO (PER SERVING)
CALORIES 364, **FAT** 25.3g, **PROTEIN** 19.2g, **CARBS** 6.5g, **FIBER** 1.8g

CHEESY BROCCOLI AND HAM CASSEROLE

1 tablespoon extra-virgin olive oil

1 (14-ounce) package riced cauliflower

¼ cup diced onion

12 ounces chopped broccoli florets

3 large eggs

⅓ cup heavy whipping cream

2 teaspoons salt

1 teaspoon black pepper

1 tablespoon dried parsley

1 teaspoon smoked paprika

1 teaspoon dry mustard

1 teaspoon onion powder

1 teaspoon garlic powder

2 cups diced ham

½ cup grated Parmesan cheese

1½ cups shredded cheddar cheese

MAKES 8 SERVINGS

This simple-to-prepare casserole is versatile enough to be served for lunch, dinner, or a Sunday brunch.

PREHEAT the oven to 350°F. Have a 9- by 13-inch baking dish ready.

IN a large skillet over medium heat, heat the olive oil. Add the riced cauliflower and onion and cook, stirring, until soft, 3 to 5 minutes. Set aside.

IN a microwave-safe bowl, heat the broccoli in the microwave oven for 5 minutes. Set aside.

IN a medium bowl, whisk the eggs until frothy. Add the cream, salt, pepper, parsley, paprika, dry mustard, onion powder, and garlic powder and mix until combined. Add the ham, Parmesan cheese, and 1 cup of the cheddar cheese and mix to combine.

ADD the egg mixture and broccoli to the cauliflower mixture and mix well. Pour the mixture into the baking dish and top with the remaining ½ cup cheddar cheese.

BAKE for 30 minutes, or until the casserole is bubbly and the cheese is golden brown. Serve hot.

NUTRITIONAL INFO (PER SERVING)
CALORIES 182, **FAT** 18.6g, **PROTEIN** 22.5g, **CARBS** 7.2g, **FIBER** 2.4g

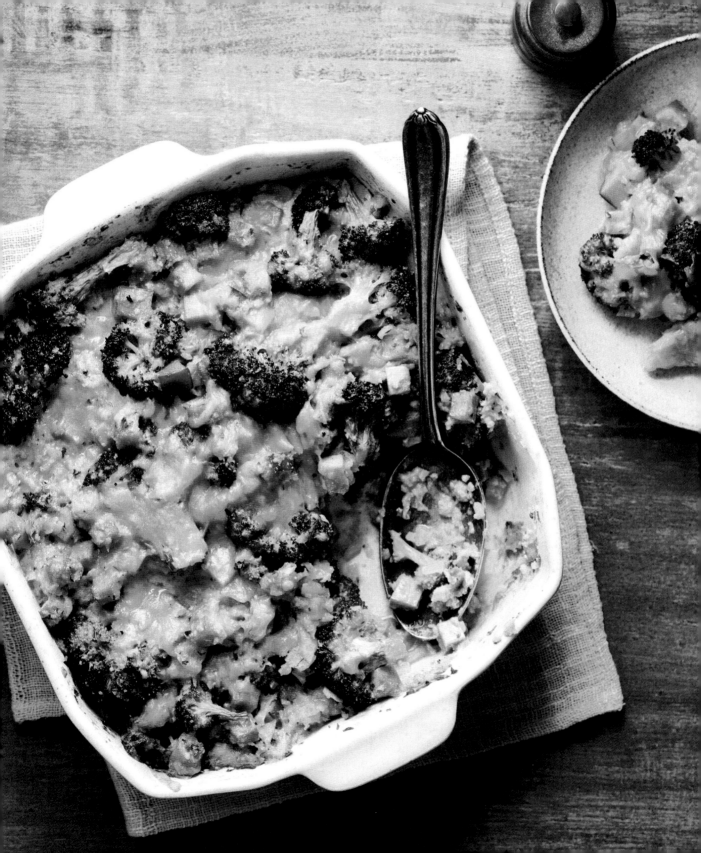

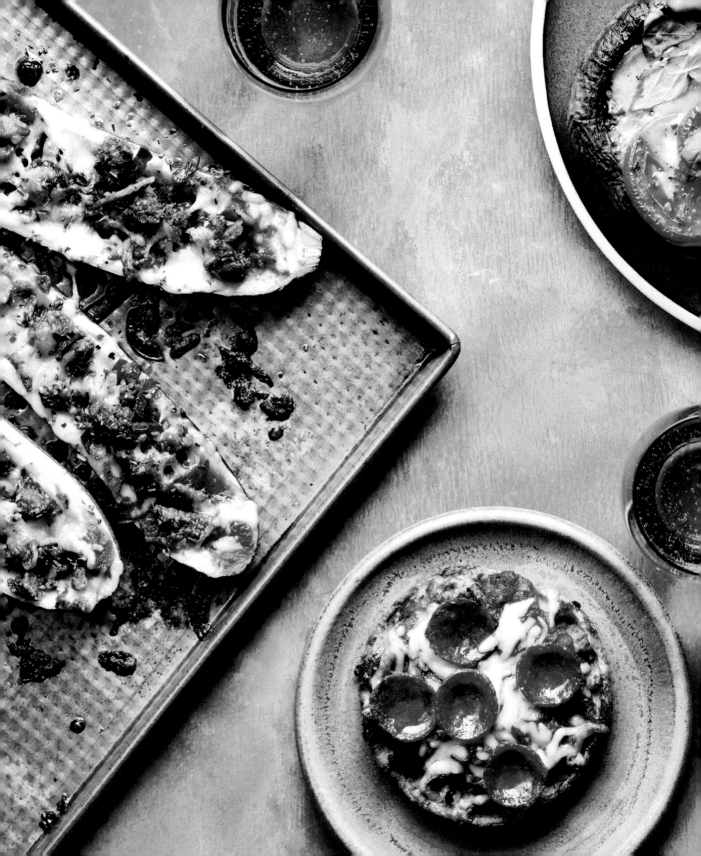

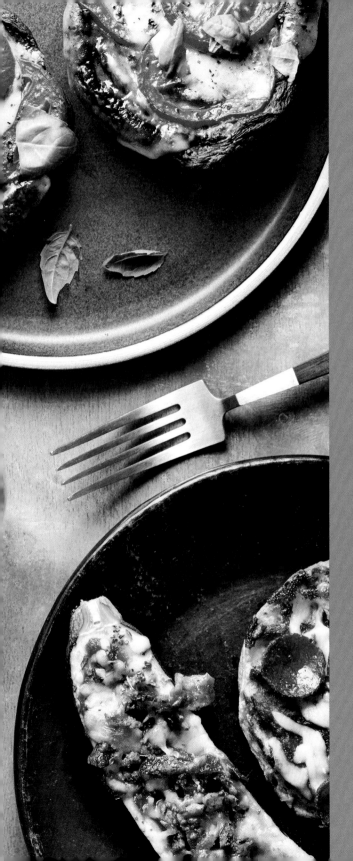

SKIP THE TAKEOUT

CHEESE-STUFFED PIZZA CRUST

1¾ cups shredded part-skim low-moisture mozzarella cheese

¾ cup blanched almond flour

2 tablespoons cream cheese

1 large egg

1 teaspoon dried rosemary, optional

12 string cheese sticks

Pizza toppings of your choice

MAKES 2 (12-INCH) PIZZA CRUSTS (6 SERVINGS EACH)
This pizza crust is absolutely amazing! I think I might make it this way all the time. I tested the recipe with many different brands and types of cheese sticks and they all work perfectly.

PREHEAT the oven to 350°F. Have a pizza pan or baking sheet and two large sheets of parchment paper ready.

IN a microwave-safe bowl, mix together the mozzarella, almond flour, and cream cheese until combined. Heat in the microwave oven for 1 minute. Add the egg and rosemary, if using, and stir until it comes together in a soft dough. Let cool for a couple of minutes.

CUT the dough into two equal pieces. Place one piece on a sheet of parchment paper. Place the second piece of parchment paper over the dough. Using a rolling pin or your hands over the parchment, roll or press out the dough into the shape of your pizza pan. Place 6 cheese sticks around the outside of the dough and wrap the dough around them.

TRANSFER the rolled out dough along with the parchment paper onto the pizza pan and bake for 12 to 15 minutes, until golden brown.

ADD the toppings of your choice and bake for another 5 to 10 minutes, until the toppings have browned and are heated through. Cut into six slices and serve warm.

REPEAT to make the second pizza.

NUTRITIONAL INFO (PER SERVING)
CALORIES 199, **FAT** 9.9g, **PROTEIN** 12.3g, **CARBS** 5.3g, **FIBER** 0.8g

Note: You can store the unbaked rolled-out dough in the freezer for up to 3 months. I usually make three batches at a time to freeze six pizza crusts. I roll it out and place each rolled-out dough between two sheets of parchment paper, then lay it flat in the freezer. When you freeze it this way, it only takes about 10 minutes to completely defrost the pizza dough before you use it.

CLUB PIZZA WITH COLD RANCH SALAD

Basic Fathead Dough
(page 272; 2 unbaked
dough rounds)

¼ cup Rao's marinara sauce

1½ cups shredded part-skim
low-moisture mozzarella
cheese

½ cup crumbled Makin'
Bacon (page 270)

2 cups chopped romaine
lettuce

¼ cup diced tomatoes

½ cup shredded fresh basil

¼ cup Homemade Ranch
Salad Dressing (page 279)
or store-bought

1 avocado, thinly sliced

MAKES 2 PIZZAS (16 SERVINGS)

This recipe tastes a lot like a pizza I used to get at California Pizza Kitchen—I'm so excited to have a keto version of what was one of my favorite pizzas. If you would rather have white sauce instead of red, use Basic Condensed Cream Soup (page 266) instead of the marinara.

PREHEAT the oven to 350°F. Line a baking sheet with parchment paper or a silicone mat.

PLACE the dough rounds on the baking sheet and bake them for 12 to 15 minutes, until golden brown.

SPREAD a thin layer of marinara sauce over each crust. Sprinkle the mozzarella cheese over the crusts and top with the crumbled bacon. Bake for about 5 minutes, or until the cheese is fully melted.

IN a bowl, toss together the lettuce, tomatoes, basil, and ranch dressing. Top the pizzas with the lettuce mixture and arrange the sliced avocado over the top.

CUT each pizza into eight slices. Serve immediately.

NUTRITIONAL INFO (PER SERVING)
CALORIES 117, **FAT** 5.1g, **PROTEIN** 9.8g, **CARBS** 5g, **FIBER** 1.9g

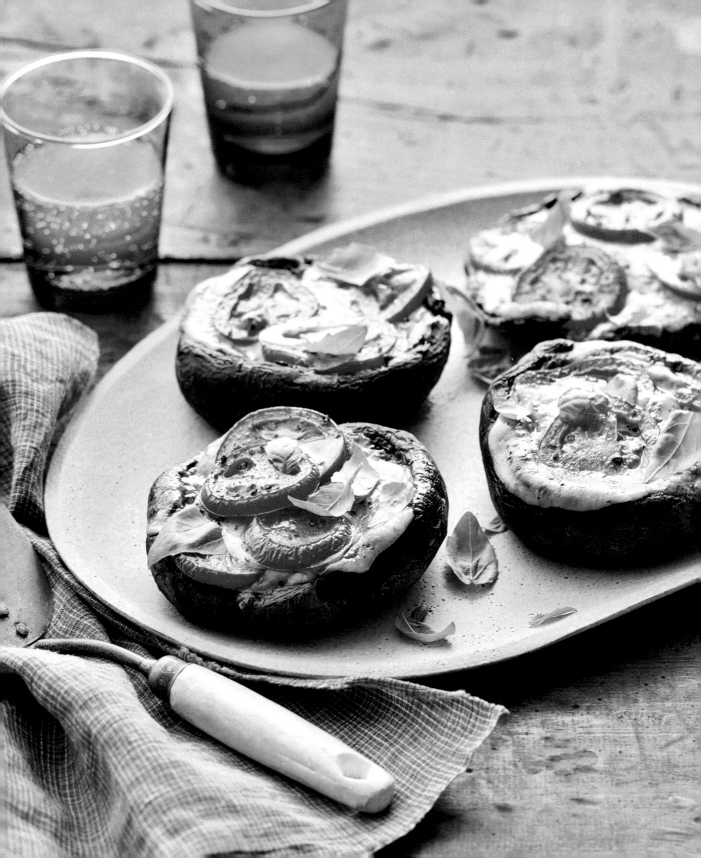

STUFFED PORTOBELLO MUSHROOM TOPS

4 ounces cream cheese, at room temperature

2 tablespoons chopped fresh basil, plus more for topping

1 tablespoon Italian seasoning

1 teaspoon smoked paprika

1 teaspoon onion powder

1 teaspoon garlic powder

1 teaspoon smoked salt (or pink Himalayan salt)

½ teaspoon black pepper, plus more if desired

4 portobello mushroom caps, cleaned and stems removed

8 slices provolone cheese

1 Roma tomato, cut into slices

Salt, optional

MAKES 4 SERVINGS

Mushrooms are fantastic for their nutritional value and low calories, and they are super filling for an entrée or side dish. We serve them typically as the "main event" of our meals, usually as a meat replacement. I also love adding a little extra fatty goodness to the stuffing with some crumbled cooked bacon.

PREHEAT the oven to 425°F. Line a baking sheet with aluminum foil.

IN a small bowl, whisk together the cream cheese, basil, Italian seasoning, smoked paprika, onion powder, garlic powder, smoked salt, and pepper until smooth.

SPREAD the cream cheese mixture equally in the mushroom caps and top each one with two slices of provolone cheese. Place a slice of tomato over the provolone. Lightly season with salt and pepper, if desired. Cover the baking sheet loosely with aluminum foil and bake for 25 to 30 minutes, until the mushrooms are tender. Sprinkle torn basil leaves over the top and serve.

NUTRITIONAL INFO (PER SERVING)
CALORIES 321, **FAT** 25.3g, **PROTEIN** 18.1g, **CARBS** 7g, **FIBER** 1.5g

PIZZA CHAFFLES

1 large egg

½ teaspoon Italian seasoning

½ cup plus 2 teaspoons shredded part-skim low-moisture mozzarella cheese, plus more for the topping

2 tablespoons Rao's homemade pizza sauce

Sliced pepperoni or any of your favorite toppings, optional

MAKES 2 SERVINGS

Who would have thought that these little pizza waffles would be one of the most popular chaffle recipes I've shared to date? They are really easy to make and amazingly delicious. The flavors actually improve if you make them ahead of time and eat them the next day. In addition to the microwave, you can reheat them in an air fryer, toaster oven, or regular oven. I love to use mini pepperonis as toppings. Sprinkling a little extra cheese in the waffle maker before adding the batter results in a crispier chaffle. Try it!

PREHEAT a mini waffle maker according to the manufacturer's instructions.

IN a small bowl, whisk together the egg and Italian seasoning. Add the ½ cup mozzarella cheese and mix until combined.

SPRINKLE 1 teaspoon mozzarella into the waffle maker and let it cook for 30 seconds. Add half the batter and cook until golden brown and crispy, about 4 minutes. Transfer the chaffle to a microwave-safe plate. Repeat with the remaining 1 teaspoon mozzarella and batter.

TOP each chaffle with 1 tablespoon pizza sauce, additional shredded mozzarella, and pepperoni, if using. Heat in the microwave for about 20 seconds and serve immediately.

NUTRITIONAL INFO (PER SERVING)
CALORIES 106, **FAT** 6.7g, **PROTEIN** 8.5g, **CARBS** 2.7g, **FIBER** 0.3g

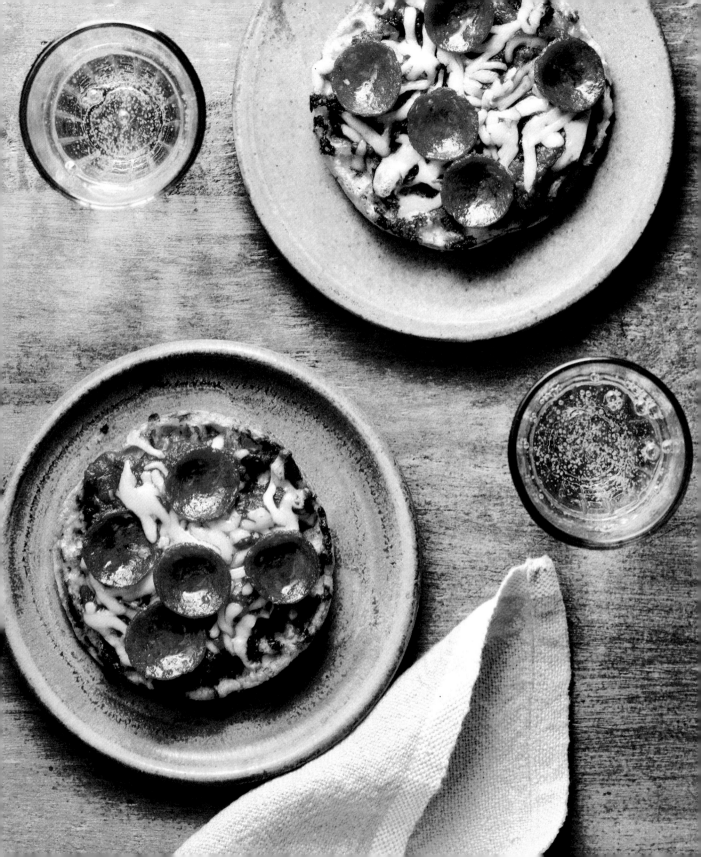

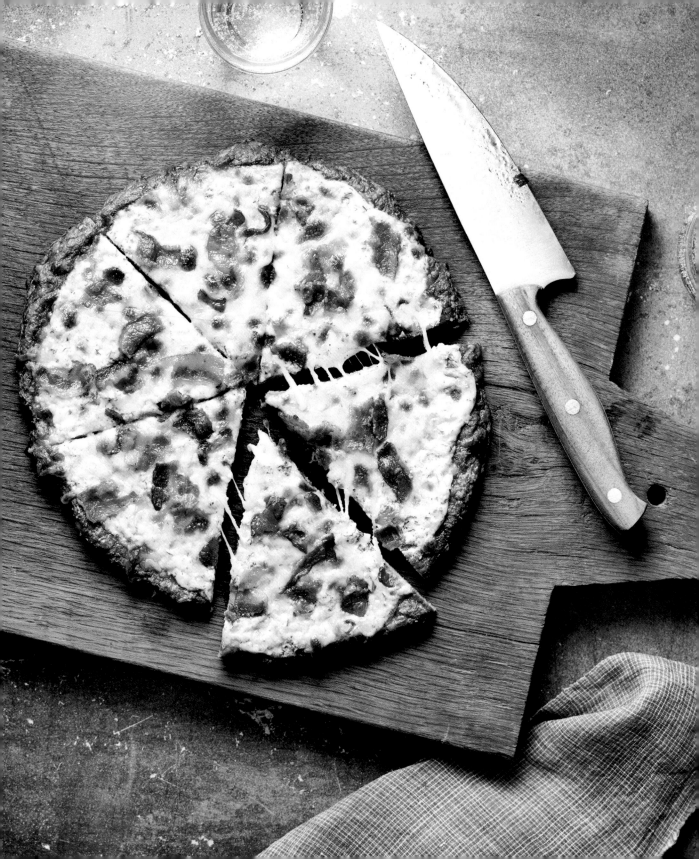

BACON-RANCH CHICKEN-CRUST PIZZA

CHICKEN CRUST

1 pound ground chicken

½ cup shredded part-skim low-moisture mozzarella cheese

1 teaspoon salt

1 teaspoon garlic powder

1 teaspoon onion powder

RANCH DRESSING

1 cup sour cream

1 tablespoon chopped fresh parsley

1 tablespoon garlic powder

1 tablespoon onion powder

1 teaspoon dried dill

1 teaspoon dried chives

1 teaspoon salt

½ teaspoon black pepper

TOPPINGS

1 cup shredded part-skim low-moisture mozzarella cheese

2 slices Makin' Bacon (page 270), diced

MAKES 6 SERVINGS

If you love chicken bacon ranch pizza, then you are going to absolutely love this low-carb version that uses ground chicken as the crust. There is no flour of any kind in this pizza.

FOR THE CHICKEN CRUST

PREHEAT the oven to 375°F. Have a baking sheet and two large sheets of parchment paper ready.

IN a large bowl, mix together the chicken, mozzarella, salt, garlic powder, and onion powder. Form into a ball and place on one sheet of parchment paper. Place the second sheet of parchment over the dough and, using a rolling pin, roll out to a round about ½ inch thick.

PLACE the rolled out dough along with the parchment paper on the baking sheet. Bake for 20 to 25 minutes, until the crust is golden brown.

FOR THE RANCH DRESSING

IN a bowl, mix together the sour cream, parsley, garlic powder, onion powder, dill, chives, salt, and pepper. Spread about 2 tablespoons of the dressing over the pizza crust, leaving ½- to ¾-inch uncovered around the edge. (Leftover ranch dressing can be stored in a covered container in the refrigerator for up to 7 days and used in salads or as a dipping sauce.) Sprinkle with the mozzarella and top with the bacon.

BAKE for 10 to 15 minutes, until the cheese has melted. Adjust the oven to broil and broil for 1 to 2 minutes, until the crust has browned and the cheese is golden brown. Cut into six slices and serve.

NUTRITIONAL INFO (PER SERVING)
CALORIES 291, **FAT** 19.4g, **PROTEIN** 22.4g, **CARBS** 6.9g, **FIBER** 0.4g

CHEESE-CRUSTED ZUCCHINI FRIES

2 large eggs

¾ cup grated Parmesan cheese

½ cup pork panko or crushed pork rinds

1 teaspoon salt

1 teaspoon dried parsley

¼ teaspoon onion powder

¼ teaspoon black pepper

⅛ teaspoon cayenne pepper

3 zucchini, cut in half and then into 4 spears each

Homemade Ranch Salad Dressing (page 279), for serving

MAKES 8 SERVINGS

I love making zucchini fries! They make a fabulous snack or side dish. If you like extra-crispy fries, just pop them in the air fryer for about 3 minutes after they're done baking.

PREHEAT the oven to 425°F. Line a baking sheet with aluminum foil and spray with nonstick cooking spray.

IN a small bowl, whisk the eggs. In a medium bowl, mix together the Parmesan, pork panko, salt, parsley, onion powder, black pepper, and cayenne.

DIP the zucchini spears into the eggs and then in the Parmesan mixture and place on the baking sheet. Bake for 20 to 23 minutes, until golden brown. Serve with ranch dressing on the side for dipping.

STORE leftovers in a covered container in the refrigerator for up to 4 days. Reheat in a toaster oven or air fryer for 3 minutes.

NUTRITIONAL INFO (PER SERVING)
CALORIES 385, **FAT** 23g, **PROTEIN** 40.7g, **CARBS** 1.3g, **FIBER** 0.3g

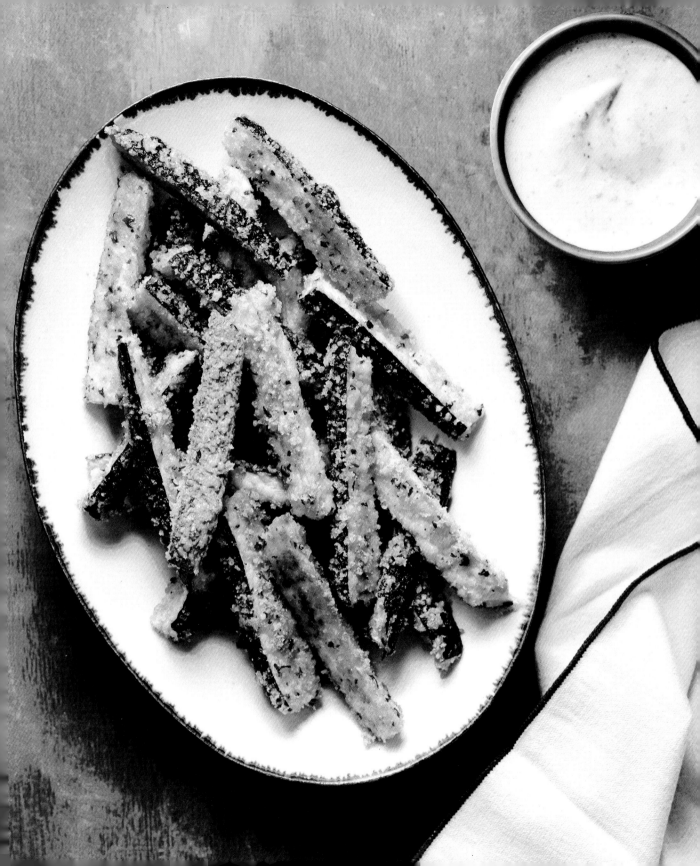

RUTABAGA FRIES

2 rutabaga, peeled and cut into ¼-inch-thick fries

3 tablespoons extra-virgin olive oil

2 tablespoons grated Parmesan cheese

1 teaspoon salt

1 teaspoon dried parsley

½ teaspoon chili powder

¼ teaspoon paprika

¼ teaspoon garlic powder

¼ teaspoon ground cumin

¼ teaspoon onion powder

¼ teaspoon black pepper

⅛ teaspoon cayenne pepper

MAKES 8 SERVINGS

Yes, you can have fries alongside your favorite burger. Rutabaga fries are soft and tender and loaded with flavor. I think you'll love them.

PREHEAT the oven to 425°F. Line a baking sheet with parchment paper or a silicone mat.

IN a medium bowl, mix together the rutabaga and olive oil until evenly coated.

IN a small bowl, mix together the Parmesan, salt, parsley, chili powder, paprika, garlic powder, cumin, onion powder, black pepper, and cayenne pepper. Sprinkle over the fries and toss until evenly coated.

SPREAD the fries out evenly on the baking sheet, making sure they aren't touching each other. Bake for 30 minutes, flipping them halfway through the baking time, until tender and crispy.

FOR extra-crispy fries, pop them in a toaster oven or air fryer for about 3 minutes.

STORE leftovers in a covered container in the refrigerator for up to 4 days. Reheat in the toaster oven or air fryer for 3 minutes, or until crispy.

NUTRITIONAL INFO (PER SERVING)
CALORIES 66, **FAT** 5.7g, **PROTEIN** 1g, **CARBS** 3.5g, **FIBER** 1g

CHICKEN PARMESAN CASSEROLE

2 tablespoons extra-virgin olive oil

3 pounds boneless skinless chicken breasts, cut into 1-inch pieces

1 tablespoon Italian seasoning

1 tablespoon onion powder

1½ teaspoons salt

1½ teaspoons black pepper

½ teaspoon red pepper flakes, optional

1 cup Rao's marinara sauce

1 cup pork panko or crushed pork rinds

1 cup grated Parmesan cheese

1 cup shredded part-skim low-moisture mozzarella cheese

1 teaspoon dried basil

MAKES 4 SERVINGS

For many people, eating keto is the best thing they've ever done. However, they still miss certain foods and chicken Parmesan is often one of them. The bread coating on the chicken and the pasta are far from being keto friendly. Here you get all those wonderful flavors without the guilt.

PREHEAT the oven to 350°F.

IN a cast-iron skillet over medium heat, heat the olive oil. Add the chicken and sprinkle with the Italian seasoning, onion powder, salt, and pepper and cook, stirring, until the chicken is almost cooked through. Add the red pepper flakes, if using, and the marinara sauce and stir to combine.

SPRINKLE with the pork panko, Parmesan, mozzarella, and basil. Transfer to the oven and bake for 15 minutes, until the cheese is melted. Adjust the oven to broil and broil for 5 minutes, until the cheese is golden brown. Serve warm.

NUTRITIONAL INFO (PER SERVING)
CALORIES 458, **FAT** 21.8g, **PROTEIN** 51.4g, **CARBS** 10.3g, **FIBER** 1.8g

Note: *If you don't have a cast-iron skillet, cook the chicken in a regular skillet and transfer the mixture to an 8-inch square baking dish after you've mixed the chicken with marinara and seasonings. Top with the pork panko, Parmesan, mozzarella, and basil and bake for 20 minutes, or until the cheese is melted. Adjust the oven to broil and broil for 3 to 5 minutes, until the cheese is golden brown.*

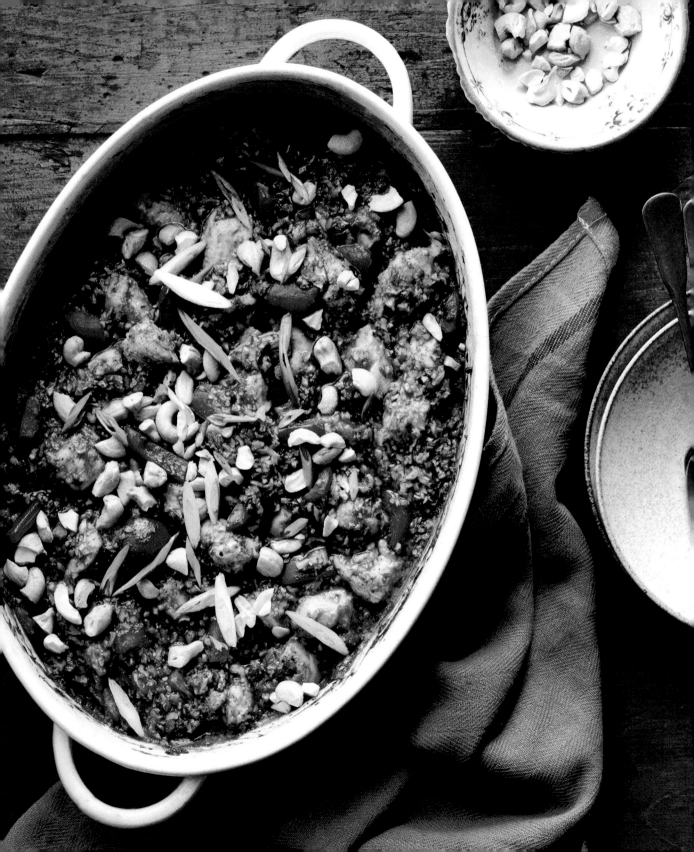

CASHEW CHICKEN WITH CAULIFLOWER RICE

CHICKEN

1 pound boneless skinless chicken breasts, cut into 1-inch pieces

1 (10-ounce) bag riced cauliflower

1 red bell pepper, chopped

1 teaspoon salt

½ teaspoon black pepper

SAUCE

½ cup coconut aminos or soy sauce

2 tablespoons Sukrin Gold brown sugar sweetener

2 tablespoons extra-virgin olive oil

1 tablespoon sriracha

1 tablespoon cashew butter or almond butter

1 tablespoon apple cider vinegar

2 teaspoons minced garlic

1 teaspoon coconut aminos garlic sauce or 1 teaspoon minced garlic

1 teaspoon xanthan gum

¼ cup chopped cashews

Sliced green onion, optional

MAKES 6 SERVINGS

Coconut aminos garlic sauce, another low-sodium soy-free substitute for soy sauce, is loaded with minerals, vitamins, and 17 amino acids. It's got a really nice garlic flavor to it. Broccoli is a nice substitute for the red pepper, but it will add about 5 minutes to the cook time.

FOR THE CHICKEN

PREHEAT the oven to 375°F.

MIX together the chicken, cauliflower, bell pepper, salt, pepper, and ¼ cup water in a 9- by 13-inch baking dish and bake for 10 minutes. Drain any excess liquid.

FOR THE SAUCE

IN a saucepan over medium heat, whisk together the coconut aminos, sweetener, olive oil, sriracha, cashew butter, vinegar, garlic, coconut aminos garlic sauce, xanthan gum, and ½ cup water. Cook until the mixture starts to bubble.

POUR the sauce over the chicken mixture and stir until the ingredients are fully coated. Bake for 10 minutes, or until the chicken is completely done and the vegetables are tender. Sprinkle with chopped cashews and sliced green onion, if using, and serve warm.

NUTRITIONAL INFO (PER SERVING)
CALORIES 136, **FAT** 8.3g, **PROTEIN** 9.3g, **CARBS** 7.4g, **FIBER** 1.8g

HASSELBACK CAJUN CHICKEN

2 tablespoons extra-virgin olive oil

2 tablespoons Cajun seasoning

2 teaspoons garlic powder

1½ teaspoons dried oregano

3 (3-ounce) boneless skinless chicken breasts

⅓ green bell pepper, thinly sliced

⅓ red bell pepper, thinly sliced

⅓ yellow bell pepper, thinly sliced

½ cup thinly sliced white onion

6 slices provolone cheese

Chopped fresh parsley, for garnish

MAKES 3 SERVINGS

I love this method of making several deep cuts into chicken breasts and stuffing them with your choice of ingredients. Not only is it completely delicious, it looks impressive enough to serve at a dinner party. The same method can be used for other meats such as pork roast or steak, and for vegetables such as butternut squash, red and green peppers, tomatoes, and artichokes.

PREHEAT the oven to 400°F. Lightly grease a baking dish.

IN a large bowl, mix together the olive oil, Cajun seasoning, garlic powder, and oregano. Add the chicken and stir to coat completely. Marinate for 10 minutes.

CUT five or six slits in each chicken breast, making sure not to cut all the way through. Stuff each slit with equal amounts of green, red, and yellow bell peppers; onion; and provolone cheese.

PLACE the breasts in the baking dish and bake for 25 to 30 minutes, until the chicken is cooked through. Serve hot.

(continued)

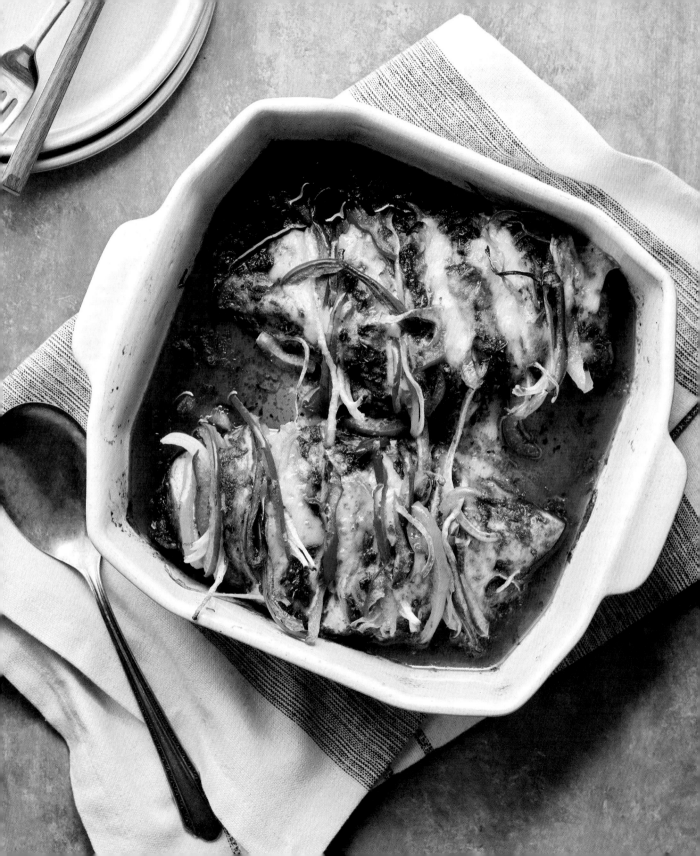

VARIATIONS

Instead of peppers, onions, and provolone, stuff the chicken with:

Spinach and goat cheese

Bacon and cheese

Ham and cheese with tomatoes

Black Forest ham and cheddar

Gouda and spinach

Sausage and Colby Jack cheese

Pesto and ham

Spinach and ricotta

Tomato, basil, and mozzarella

Zucchini, spinach, and tomato

Tomatoes, olives, and pesto

NUTRITIONAL INFO (PER SERVING)
CALORIES 376, **FAT** 25.1g, **PROTEIN** 28.2g, **CARBS** 9.8g, **FIBER** 1.9g

TACO CHAFFLES

FILLING

1 pound ground beef

1 teaspoon chili powder

1 teaspoon ground cumin

½ teaspoon garlic powder

½ teaspoon cocoa powder, optional

½ teaspoon smoked paprika

¼ teaspoon onion powder

¼ teaspoon salt

CHAFFLES

2 large eggs

1 cup shredded cheddar cheese or part-skim low-moisture mozzarella cheese mozzarella

½ teaspoon Italian seasoning

TOPPINGS

Shredded lettuce

Chopped tomatoes

Shredded cheddar cheese

MAKES 4 SERVINGS

Taco Tuesday has just become keto approved with the creation of the chaffle, a waffle made with cheese. The cocoa powder in the filling is optional but it really enhances the flavors of all the other seasonings so I highly recommend using it. It's so easy to make your own taco seasoning that there's no real reason to purchase the premade packets, which are loaded with not-so-good additives and preservatives. I like to make a double or triple batch so I always have some seasoning on hand.

FOR THE FILLING

IN a large skillet over medium heat, cook the ground beef, breaking it up with a wooden spoon, until cooked through. Add the chili powder, cumin, garlic powder, cocoa powder (if using), paprika, onion powder, and salt and stir to combine.

FOR THE CHAFFLES

PREHEAT a mini waffle maker according to the manufacturer's instructions.

IN a small bowl, whisk the eggs. Add the cheese and Italian seasoning and mix until combined. Pour one-fourth of the batter into the waffle maker and cook for 3 to 4 minutes, until golden. Drape the chaffle over a skewer or wooden spoon handle suspended over two glasses and let rest. As it cools it will stay in a taco shape. Repeat with the rest of the batter to make four chaffles.

DIVIDE the filling between the chaffles, top with lettuce, tomatoes, and cheese and serve warm.

NUTRITIONAL INFO (PER SERVING)
CALORIES 219, **FAT** 9.6g, **PROTEIN** 30g, **CARBS** 1.9g, **FIBER** 0.6g

Note: *The seasoning can be stored in a covered container at room temperature for up to 6 months. I keep mine in small mason jars in my kitchen pantry. Just add a label to it and you are good to go. To use, add 4 teaspoons of the spice mixture for every 1 pound of ground beef.*

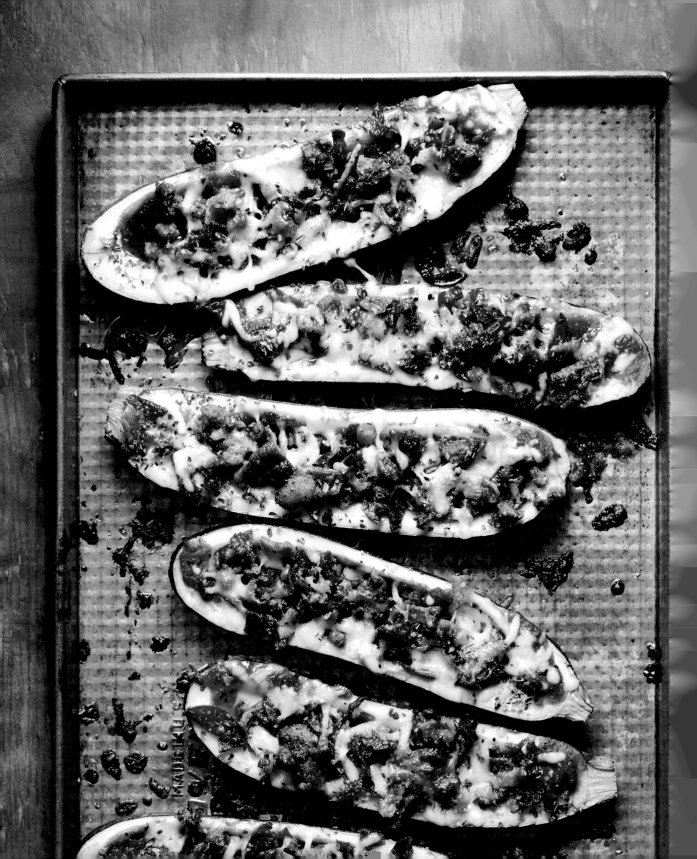

STUFFED ZUCCHINI BOATS

3 zucchini, cut lengthwise in half

6 tablespoons Rao's marinara sauce

2 teaspoons Italian seasoning

3 tablespoons chopped pepperoni

3 tablespoons cooked crumbled sausage

3 tablespoons crumbled Makin' Bacon (page 270)

¼ cup shredded part-skim low-moisture mozzarella cheese

¼ teaspoon dried oregano

MAKES 6 SERVINGS

Here is a dish your kids will think is really fun, with a filling that tastes like pizza and a bowl they can eat.

PREHEAT the oven to 400°F.

SCOOP out a shallow indentation in each zucchini with a spoon to make a boat, and discard the filling. Place the zucchini on a microwave-safe plate and heat in the microwave for 2 minutes to soften. Use a paper towel to soak up any moisture.

IN a small bowl, mix together the marinara sauce and Italian seasoning. Spread 1 tablespoon into each indentation. Top with layers of pepperoni, sausage, and bacon. Sprinkle with the cheese and oregano.

BAKE for 15 minutes, or until the cheese has melted. Serve hot.

NUTRITIONAL INFO (PER SERVING)
CALORIES 187, **FAT** 13.6g, **PROTEIN** 12g, **CARBS** 4g, **FIBER** 0.7g

OVEN-BAKED GARLIC PARMESAN RIBS

RIBS AND RUB

1 rack baby back ribs, cut in half

1 tablespoon extra-virgin olive oil

1 tablespoon dried oregano

2 teaspoons salt

1 teaspoon black pepper

GARLIC-PARMESAN SAUCE

1 cup grated Parmesan cheese

8 tablespoons butter, melted

6 garlic cloves, minced

1 tablespoon chopped fresh parsley

MAKES 4 SERVINGS

I've made ribs in the slow cooker, in an Instant Pot, and on the grill, but there are some days that I love to just pop them in the oven and roast them. With a simple rub for the ribs and a cheesy garlic sauce, these will definitely hit the spot.

PREHEAT the oven to 350°F. Line a baking sheet with aluminum foil.

FOR THE RIBS AND RUB

REMOVE the membrane from the back of the ribs with a sharp knife. Pat the ribs dry with paper towels. Drizzle with olive oil, sprinkle with the oregano, salt, and pepper and massage them into the ribs. Place the ribs on the baking sheet, cover with aluminum foil, and bake for 1 hour, until tender.

FOR THE SAUCE

IN a small bowl, mix together the Parmesan, melted butter, garlic, and parsley.

REMOVE the foil and brush the garlic butter sauce over the ribs. Return the ribs to the oven and bake for an additional 10 minutes. Ribs are considered done when the internal temperature reaches 145°F, but if you let them get to an internal temp of 190 to 203°F, the collagens and fats melt, making them more tender and juicy. Serve warm.

NUTRITIONAL INFO (PER SERVING)
CALORIES 349, **FAT** 33.1g, **PROTEIN** 10g, **CARBS** 4.7g, **FIBER** 0.8g

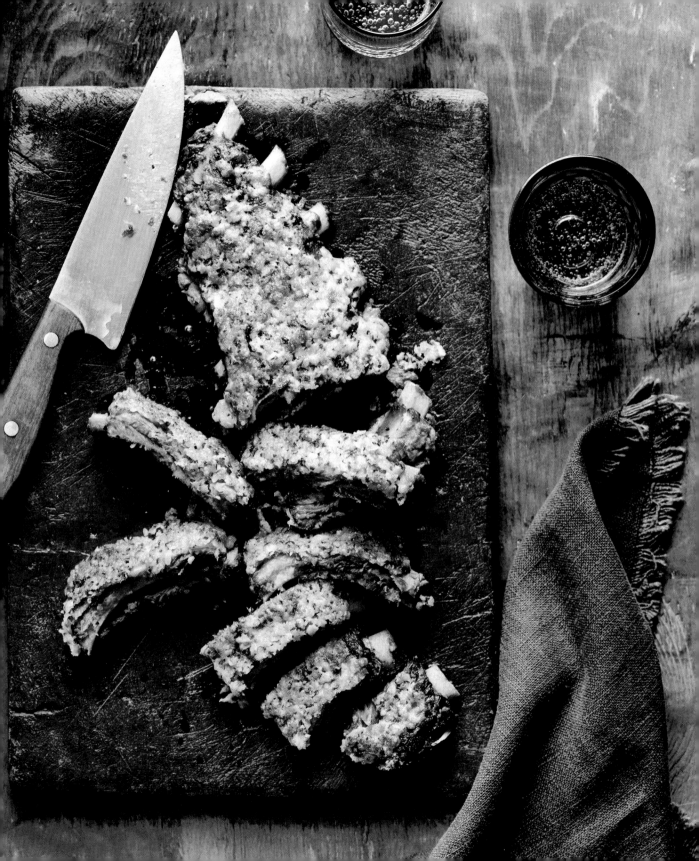

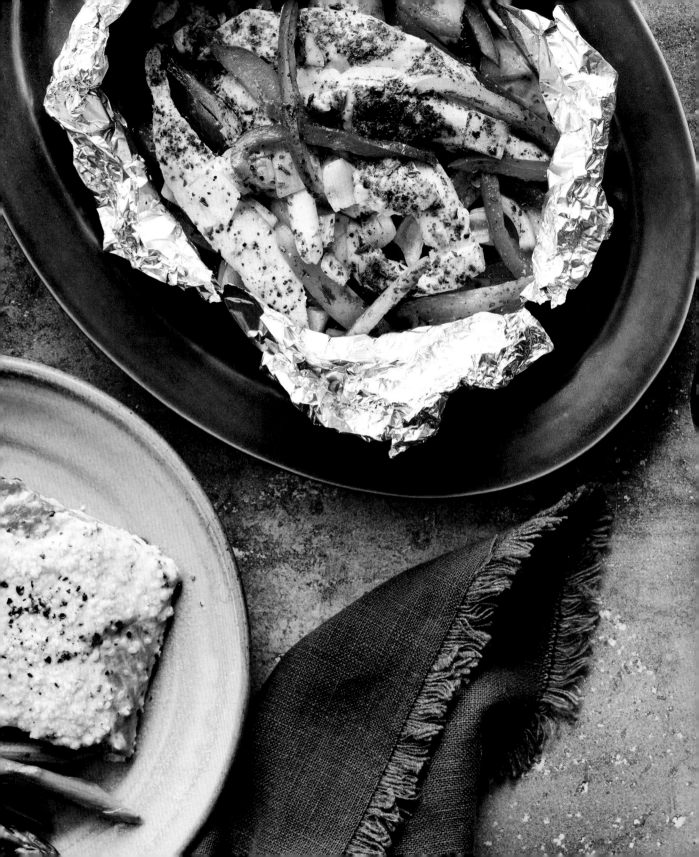

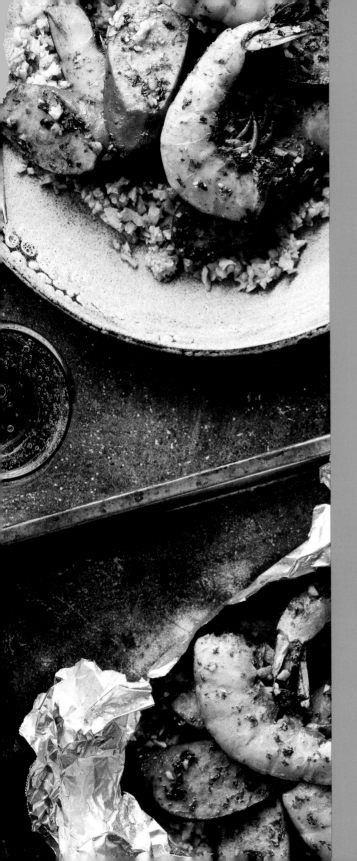

OVEN-BAKED FOIL PACKS

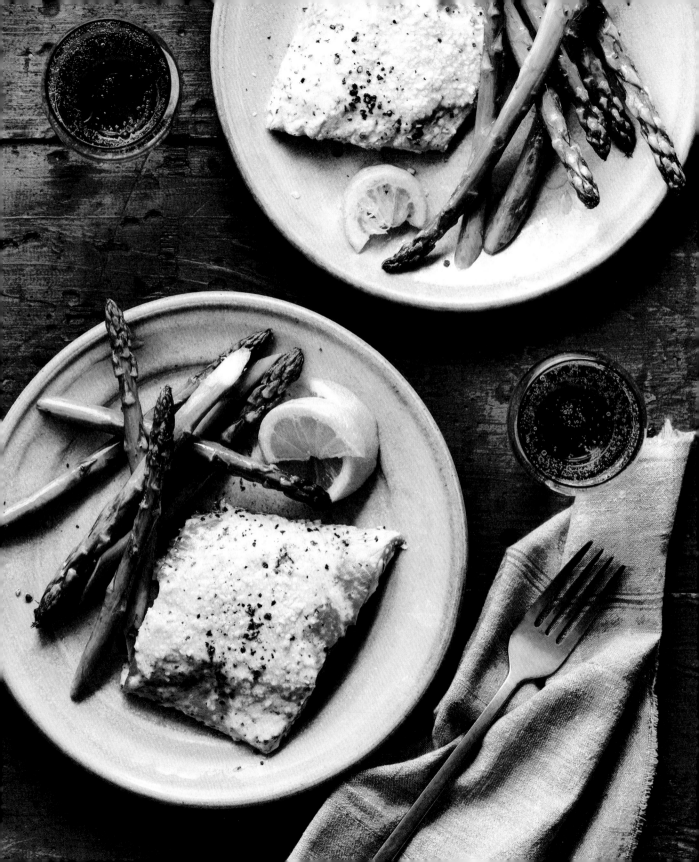

SIMPLE SAVORY SALMON FOIL PACK

½ cup chopped asparagus or 6 whole spears

2 tablespoons extra-virgin olive oil

1 (5-ounce) salmon fillet

1 tablespoon mayonnaise

1 teaspoon lemon juice

1 teaspoon Italian seasoning

2 tablespoons grated Parmesan cheese

½ teaspoon salt

MAKES 1 SERVING

Never has salmon tasted so good or been made as quickly as baking it in a foil pack. The asparagus pairs nicely with the salmon and makes this a well-balanced, complete meal.

PREHEAT the oven to 350°F. Have a large sheet of aluminum foil and a large baking sheet ready.

PLACE the asparagus in the center of the foil and drizzle with 1 tablespoon of the olive oil. Place the salmon, skin side down, on top of the asparagus.

IN a small bowl, combine the mayonnaise, lemon juice, Italian seasoning, and remaining 1 tablespoon olive oil. Spread the mixture over the salmon and sprinkle with the Parmesan cheese and salt.

POUR 1 teaspoon water into the bottom of the foil pack, fold up the foil, and seal the pack. Place the foil pack on the baking sheet and bake for about 20 minutes, or until the salmon reaches an internal temperature of 145°F.

NUTRITIONAL INFO (PER SERVING)
CALORIES 576, **FAT** 47.8g, **PROTEIN** 36.9g, **CARBS** 3.4g, **FIBER** 1.4g

CREAMY DIJON TILAPIA FOIL PACK

1 tablespoon Dijon mustard

1 teaspoon butter, melted

1 teaspoon minced garlic

½ teaspoon horseradish sauce

½ teaspoon salt

¼ teaspoon pepper

½ cup sliced radishes

1 teaspoon extra-virgin olive oil

1 (4-ounce) tilapia fillet

1 teaspoon chopped fresh parsley

MAKES 1 SERVING

The radishes will taste like potatoes after baking. The flavors work well with other vegetables too. Try some of your favorites.

PREHEAT the oven to 350°F. Have a large sheet of aluminum foil and a large baking sheet ready.

IN a small bowl, combine the Dijon, butter, garlic, horseradish, salt, and pepper.

PLACE the radishes on the foil and drizzle with the olive oil. Place the tilapia fillet on the radishes and spread the mustard sauce over the top.

POUR 1 teaspoon water into the bottom of the foil pack, fold up the foil, and seal the pack.

PLACE the foil pack on the baking sheet and bake for 15 to 20 minutes, until the internal temperature of the tilapia reaches 145°F. Top with the parsley and serve warm.

NUTRITIONAL INFO (PER SERVING)
CALORIES 549, **FAT** 18.6g, **PROTEIN** 94g, **CARBS** 2.2g, **FIBER** 0.5g

PROSCIUTTO-WRAPPED COD FOIL PACK

½ cup chopped asparagus, or 6 whole spears

1 tablespoon extra-virgin olive oil

1 (4-ounce) cod fillet

1 tablespoon lemon juice

¼ teaspoon dried dill

¼ teaspoon onion powder

¼ teaspoon garlic powder

¼ teaspoon salt

¼ teaspoon pepper

3 ounces prosciutto

MAKES 1 SERVING

I love adding prosciutto to fish and vegetables. Not only is it super tasty but it's a wonderful healthy added fat and protein that complements fish nicely.

PREHEAT the oven to 350°F. Have a large sheet of aluminum foil and a large baking sheet ready.

PLACE the asparagus on the foil and drizzle with the olive oil. Place the cod on a plate and sprinkle with the lemon juice. Sprinkle the dill, onion powder, garlic powder, salt, and pepper over the cod. Wrap the prosciutto around the cod and place on the asparagus.

POUR 1 tablespoon water into the bottom of the foil pack, fold up the foil, and seal the pack. Place the foil pack on the baking sheet and bake for about 20 minutes, or until the internal temperature of the cod reaches 145°F.

NUTRITIONAL INFO (PER SERVING)
CALORIES 575, **FAT** 47.7g, **PROTEIN** 32.3g, **CARBS** 6.3g, **FIBER** 1.8g

FIESTA CHICKEN FOIL PACK

¼ cup julienned green bell pepper

¼ cup julienned red bell pepper

¼ cup julienned orange bell pepper

¼ cup chopped onion

1 tablespoon extra-virgin olive oil

½ teaspoon salt

¼ teaspoon black pepper

4 ounces chicken tenders, cut into ½-inch-thick strips

1 tablespoon lemon juice

1 teaspoon chili powder

1 teaspoon ground cumin

½ teaspoon dried oregano

¼ teaspoon garlic powder

MAKES 1 SERVING

The colorful vegetables make this as beautiful to look at as it is delicious to eat. It's fantastic as leftovers for the next day too.

PREHEAT the oven to 375°F. Have a large sheet of aluminum foil and a large baking sheet ready.

PLACE the green, red, and orange peppers and the onion on the foil, drizzle with the olive oil, and season with the salt and pepper.

IN a bowl, toss the chicken strips with the lemon juice, then arrange them over the vegetables. Sprinkle with the chili powder, cumin, oregano, and garlic powder.

POUR 1 teaspoon water into the bottom of the foil pack, fold up the foil, and seal the pack. Place the foil pack on the baking sheet and bake for 20 minutes, or until the chicken is fully cooked, or until the internal temperature is 165°F.

NUTRITIONAL INFO (PER SERVING)
CALORIES 327, **FAT** 18.2g, **PROTEIN** 28g, **CARBS** 14.5g, **FIBER** 4.5g

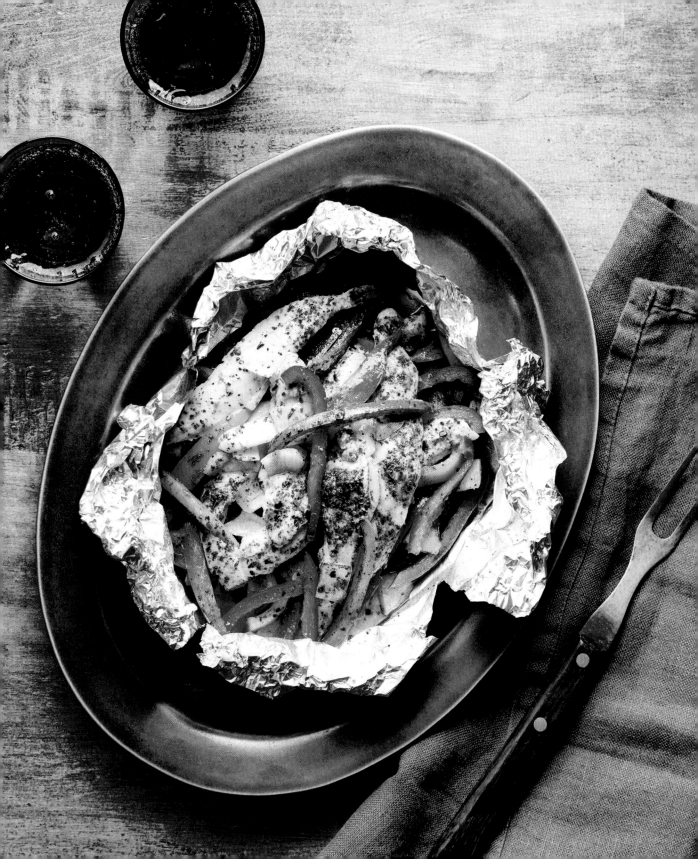

ROSEMARY CHICKEN FOIL PACK

2 tablespoons mayonnaise

1 tablespoon grated Parmesan cheese

1 teaspoon chopped fresh rosemary

1 teaspoon salt

½ teaspoon black pepper

¼ teaspoon garlic powder

1 cup thinly sliced zucchini

2 tablespoons extra-virgin olive oil

8 ounces chicken tenders

2 tablespoons shredded part-skim low-moisture mozzarella cheese

MAKES 2 SERVINGS

This is my favorite chicken foil pack recipe. I love fresh rosemary so much that I have a few rosemary plants in my yard.

PREHEAT the oven to 375°F. Have two large sheets of aluminum foil and a large baking sheet ready.

IN a small bowl, combine the mayonnaise, Parmesan cheese, rosemary, salt, pepper, and garlic powder.

DIVIDE the zucchini between the two sheets of foil and drizzle with the olive oil. Place the chicken on top of the zucchini and spread with the mayonnaise mixture. Pour 1 teaspoon water into the bottom of each of the foil packs, fold up the foil, and seal.

BAKE for 20 minutes. Open the packs, sprinkle with the mozzarella cheese, and reseal. Place the foil pack on the baking sheet and bake for another 5 minutes, or until the chicken reaches an internal temperature of 165°F.

NUTRITIONAL INFO (PER SERVING)
CALORIES 383, **FAT** 29.2g, **PROTEIN** 28.2g, **CARBS** 1.9g, **FIBER** 0.5g

BARBECUE CHICKEN FOIL PACK

3 tablespoons AlternaSweets original BBQ sauce

1 ounce cream cheese, at room temperature

1 tablespoon grated Parmesan cheese

½ cup sliced radishes

1 tablespoon extra-virgin olive oil

¼ teaspoon salt

¼ teaspoon black pepper

1 (3- to 4-ounce) skin-on chicken thigh

MAKES 1 SERVING

If you are in the mood for barbecue but don't want to leave the house, this recipe can be whipped up in no time at all. And, there's almost nothing to clean up.

PREHEAT the oven to 350°F. Have a large sheet of aluminum foil and a large baking sheet ready.

IN a small bowl, combine the BBQ sauce, cream cheese, and Parmesan cheese and mix well.

PLACE the radishes on the foil, drizzle with the olive oil, and sprinkle with the salt and pepper. Place the chicken thigh on the radishes and spread the sauce over the top.

POUR 1 teaspoon water into the bottom of the foil pack, fold up the foil, and seal the pack. Place the foil pack on the baking sheet and bake for 20 minutes, or until the chicken reaches an internal temperature of 165°F.

NUTRITIONAL INFO (PER SERVING)
CALORIES 444, **FAT** 31.3g, **PROTEIN** 33.5g, **CARBS** 9.4g, **FIBER** 0.8g

CHEESY BACON RANCH CHICKEN FOIL PACK

2 tablespoons mayonnaise

½ teaspoon dried parsley

½ teaspoon salt

¼ teaspoon garlic powder

¼ teaspoon onion powder

¼ teaspoon dried dill

¼ teaspoon black pepper

10 ounces broccoli, cut into florets

2 tablespoons extra-virgin olive oil

1 (3-ounce) boneless skinless chicken breast, cut horizontally into two thin pieces

2 tablespoons shredded part-skim low-moisture mozzarella cheese

3 tablespoons crumbled Makin' Bacon (page 270)

Chopped fresh chives, for garnish

MAKES 2 SERVINGS

This is an easy recipe to double. By cutting chicken breasts thin, they cook at the same time as the vegetables for the perfect meal.

PREHEAT the oven to 350°F. Have two large sheets of aluminum foil and a large baking sheet ready.

IN a small bowl, combine the mayonnaise, parsley, salt, garlic powder, onion powder, dill, and pepper.

PLACE half of the broccoli on each sheet of aluminum foil and drizzle with the olive oil. Place the chicken on the broccoli and spread with the mayonnaise sauce.

POUR 1 tablespoon water into the bottom of each foil pack, fold up the foil, and seal the pack. Place the foil pack on the baking sheet and bake for 20 minutes. Open the packs, sprinkle with the mozzarella cheese and bacon, and reseal. Bake for another 5 minutes, or until the chicken reaches an internal temperature of 165°F.

TOP with chives and serve warm.

NUTRITIONAL INFO (PER SERVING)
CALORIES 300, **FAT** 27.2g, **PROTEIN** 10.3g, **CARBS** 5.3g, **FIBER** 1.7g

CHIPOTLE STEAK FAJITAS FOIL PACK

MARINADE AND STEAK

1 tablespoon extra-virgin olive oil

1 tablespoon apple cider vinegar

1 tablespoon Tabasco chipotle pepper sauce

1 tablespoon minced garlic

1 teaspoon chili powder

½ teaspoon ground cumin

4 ounces flank steak, cut into ½-inch slices

FAJITAS

⅓ cup chopped green bell pepper

¼ cup chopped red bell pepper

1 teaspoon extra-virgin olive oil

½ teaspoon salt

¼ teaspoon black pepper

MAKES 1 SERVING

No need to head out for dinner when making fajitas at home is this easy. Be sure to ask your local grocery store butcher to cut the flank steak into slices, which will save you time in the kitchen. This is a good recipe to double or even quadruple.

FOR THE MARINADE AND STEAK

IN a zip-top bag, mix together the olive oil, vinegar, Tabasco, garlic, chili powder, and cumin. Add the steak, seal the bag, and marinate in the refrigerator for at least 1 hour.

FOR THE FAJITAS

PREHEAT the oven to 350°F. Have a large sheet of aluminum foil and a large baking sheet ready.

PLACE the green and red bell peppers on the foil, drizzle with the olive oil, and season with the salt and pepper. Place the steak on top of the peppers.

POUR 1 teaspoon water into the bottom of the foil pack, fold up the foil, and seal the pack. Place the foil pack on the baking sheet and bake for 20 minutes, or until the steak is fully cooked and reaches an internal temperature of 135°F.

NUTRITIONAL INFO (PER SERVING)
CALORIES 351, **FAT** 24.8g, **PROTEIN** 25.9g, **CARBS** 8.2g, **FIBER** 2.1g

PHILLY CHEESESTEAK FOIL PACK

½ cup sliced radishes

¼ cup diced green bell pepper

¼ cup chopped button mushrooms

1 tablespoon chopped onion

1 tablespoon extra-virgin olive oil

¼ teaspoon salt

¼ teaspoon black pepper

2 teaspoons Worcestershire sauce

1 teaspoon Italian seasoning

½ teaspoon smoked paprika

½ teaspoon onion powder

¼ teaspoon garlic powder

⅛ teaspoon cayenne pepper

4 ounces rib eye or sirloin steak, very thinly sliced

1 slice provolone cheese

MAKES 1 SERVING

You can use either rib eye or sirloin steak with this recipe. The key to achieving perfectly thin slices of meat is to freeze the steak for about an hour before slicing. This will make sure that the meat is firm enough to cut into very thin slices. Use a really sharp knife and cut the meat against the grain.

PREHEAT the oven to 350°F. Have a large sheet of aluminum foil and a large baking sheet ready.

PLACE the radishes, bell pepper, mushrooms, and onion on the foil, drizzle with the olive oil, and season with the salt and pepper.

IN a small bowl, mix together the Worcestershire, Italian seasoning, smoked paprika, onion powder, garlic powder, and cayenne pepper. Toss with the steak until evenly coated and arrange on the vegetables.

FOLD up the foil, seal the pack, place it on the baking sheet, and bake for 20 minutes. Open the pack, place the slice of provolone on the steak, and reseal. Bake for about 5 more minutes, or until the steak is fully cooked and reaches an internal temperature of 135°F.

NUTRITIONAL INFO (PER SERVING)
CALORIES 296, **FAT** 13g, **PROTEIN** 33g, **CARBS** 9g, **FIBER** 2g

TERIYAKI STEAK AND BROCCOLI FOIL PACK

MARINADE AND STEAK

¼ cup coconut aminos

2 tablespoons Sukrin Gold brown sugar sweetener

1 teaspoon ginger paste

1 teaspoon minced garlic

½ teaspoon xanthan gum

8 ounces flank steak, cut into ½-inch strips

1 cup chopped broccoli

2 tablespoons extra-virgin olive oil

½ teaspoon salt

2 tablespoons chopped green onion

2 teaspoons sesame seeds, optional

MAKES 2 SERVINGS

Your non-keto friends will love this recipe and they'll never know it's keto friendly. The marinade is the key to the incredible flavor.

FOR THE MARINADE AND STEAK

IN a zip-top bag, mix together the coconut aminos, sweetener, ginger paste, garlic, and xanthan gum. Add the steak and marinate for at least 1 hour.

PREHEAT the oven to 425°F. Have two large sheets of aluminum foil and a large baking sheet ready.

PLACE half of the broccoli on each sheet of foil, drizzle with the olive oil, and season with the salt. Place the steaks on the broccoli.

POUR 1 tablespoon water into the bottom of each foil pack, fold up the foil, and seal the packs. Place the foil packs on the baking sheet and bake for 15 to 20 minutes, until the steak is done and has reached an internal temperature of 135°F. Top with green onions and sesame seeds, if using, and serve.

NUTRITIONAL INFO (PER SERVING)
CALORIES 305, **FAT** 19.9g, **PROTEIN** 25.8g, **CARBS** 6.2g, **FIBER** 1.9g

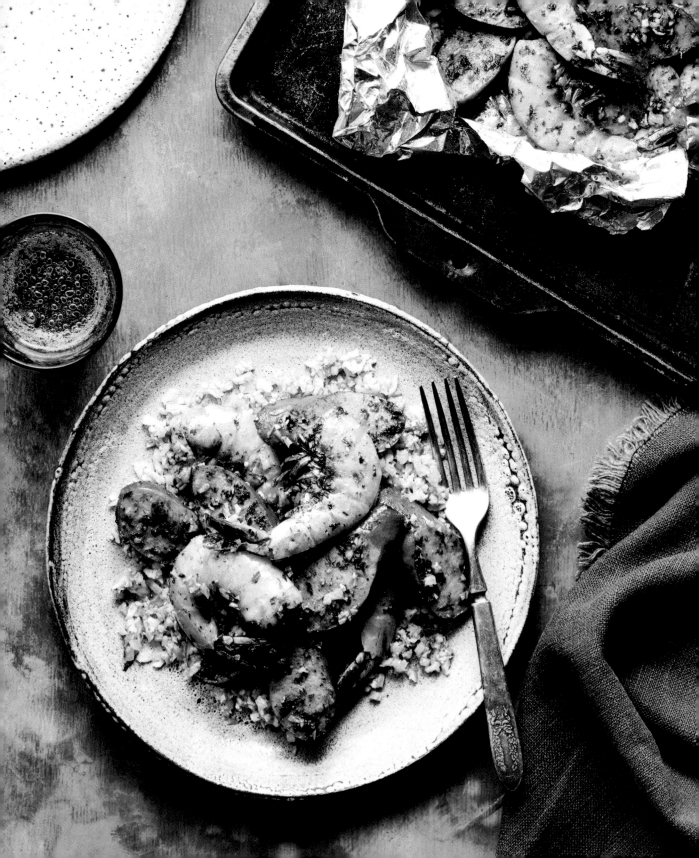

SAUSAGE AND SHRIMP FOIL PACK

2 tablespoons butter, melted

2 tablespoons extra-virgin olive oil

1 tablespoon dried parsley

1 teaspoon minced garlic

1 teaspoon Old Bay seasoning

¼ teaspoon smoked paprika

½ pound large shrimp, shelled

½ pound kielbasa sausage, cut into ½-inch-thick diagonal slices

1 cup riced cauliflower

MAKES 2 SERVINGS

For a weeknight version of surf and turf, turn to this incredibly easy recipe. It takes no time at all to throw the ingredients together and you'll have dinner on the table in about half an hour.

PREHEAT the oven to 375°F. Have two large sheets of aluminum foil and a large baking sheet ready.

IN a medium bowl, mix together the butter, olive oil, parsley, garlic, Old Bay, and smoked paprika. Add the shrimp and sausage and mix until fully coated.

PLACE half the cauliflower on each sheet of foil. Divide the shrimp and sausage mixture evenly and arrange on top of the cauliflower mixture. Fold up the foil and seal the packs.

PLACE the foil packs on the baking sheet and bake for 20 to 22 minutes, or until the shrimp is cooked through.

NUTRITIONAL INFO (PER SERVING)
CALORIES 377, **FAT** 29g, **PROTEIN** 26.8g, **CARBS** 5.7g, **FIBER** 2.2g

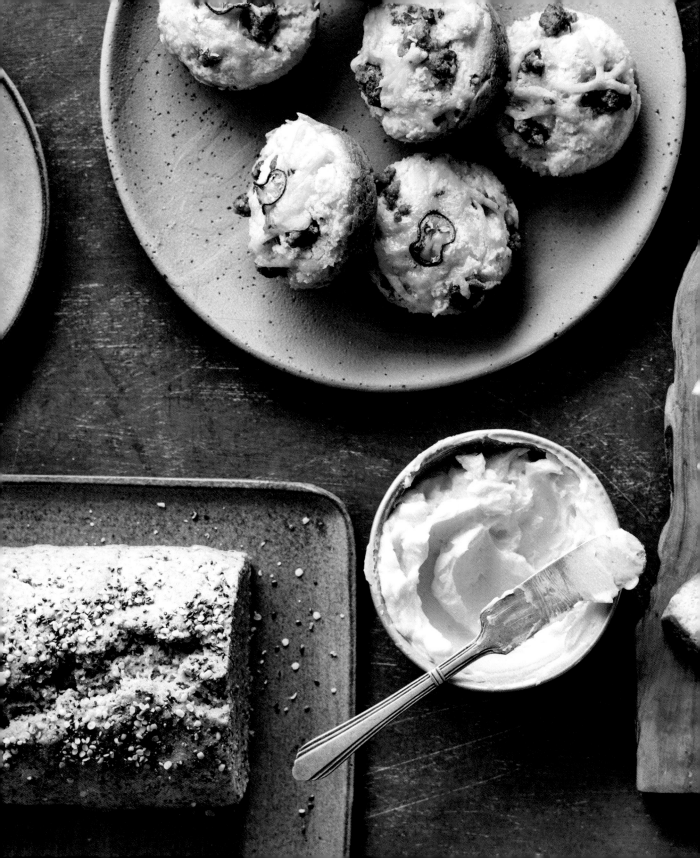

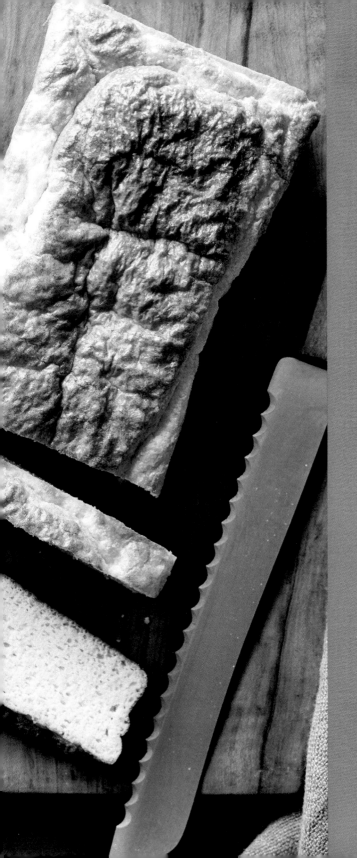

BREADS

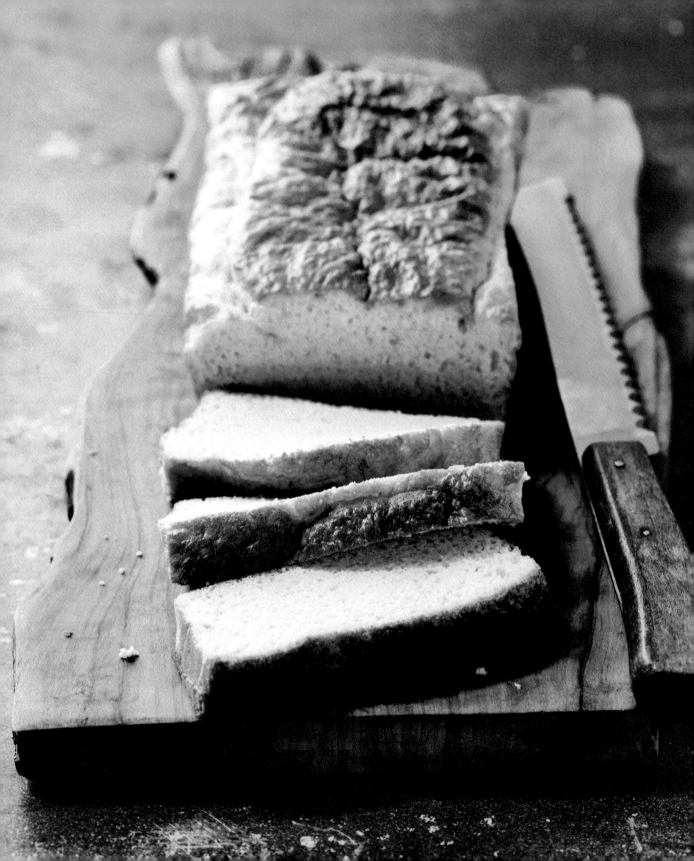

FLUFFY WHITE BREAD

8 large egg whites or 1 cup
  egg whites

½ cup cream cheese, at
  room temperature

1 cup blanched almond flour

1 teaspoon baking powder

2 tablespoons sparkling water

MAKES 1 LOAF (8 SERVINGS)

This makes a delicious, everyday bread that's great for sandwiches or toast. To shake things up, try making the bread in a waffle maker. The recipe makes enough for 4 large waffles or 8 mini waffles.

PREHEAT the oven to 350°F. Grease an 8- by 5-inch loaf pan.

IN a medium bowl using a hand mixer, beat the egg whites until they are doubled in size and soft and frothy. Add the cream cheese and continue to beat on high speed until smooth. Add the almond flour, baking powder, and sparkling water and beat on medium speed until fully combined.

POUR the batter into the prepared loaf pan. Bake for 25 to 30 minutes, until golden brown and a toothpick inserted into the center comes out clean.

NUTRITIONAL INFO (PER SERVING)
CALORIES 123, **FAT** 9.8g, **PROTEIN** 7.2g, **CARBS** 1.7g, **FIBER** 0g

MOCK WHEAT BREAD

2½ cups blanched almond flour

½ cup ground flaxseed

2 tablespoons psyllium husk

1 tablespoon baking powder

1 tablespoon unflavored collagen peptides

1 teaspoon active yeast

1 teaspoon salt

⅔ cup extra-virgin olive oil

¼ cup sour cream

7 large eggs

1 tablespoon apple cider vinegar

MAKES 1 LOAF OR 2 MINI LOAVES (20 SERVINGS)
This recipe makes a large loaf that can be sliced thin. The yeast doesn't actually do anything to the texture, but simply adds the smell of real bread. Most people taste first with their nose, so it adds a special touch. This is a hearty bread that works well for sandwiches.

PREHEAT the oven to 350°F. Grease a 9- by 5-inch loaf pan or two 6- by 3-inch mini bread loaf pans loaf pans.

IN a medium bowl, mix together the almond flour, flaxseed, psyllium husk, baking powder, collagen peptides, yeast, and salt.

IN a separate bowl, mix together the olive oil, sour cream, eggs, and vinegar. Add the almond flour mixture and mix to combine.

POUR the batter into the prepared loaf pan(s). Bake for 45 to 50 minutes for the large loaf or 38 to 40 minutes for the mini loaves, until golden brown and a toothpick inserted into the center comes out clean.

NUTRITIONAL INFO (PER SERVING)
CALORIES 197, **FAT** 13.8g, **PROTEIN** 5.2g, **CARBS** 4.4g, **FIBER** 1.7g

ALMOND BREAD

1 cup blanched almond flour

½ cup oat fiber

2 teaspoons baking powder

1 tablespoon unflavored collagen peptides

½ teaspoon salt

½ cup extra-virgin olive oil

4 large egg whites or ½ cup liquid egg whites

2 tablespoons sliced almonds, optional

MAKES 1 LOAF OR 2 MINI LOAVES (12 SERVINGS)

This recipe is one of my favorites because it not only tastes great but the collagen peptides keep it moist and bread-like. It also makes great toast.

PREHEAT the oven to 350°F. Grease a 9- by 5-inch loaf pan or two 6- by 3-inch mini loaf pans.

IN a medium bowl, mix together the almond flour, oat fiber, baking powder, collagen peptides, and salt. Add the olive oil and ½ cup water and mix until combined.

IN a separate bowl using a hand mixer, beat the egg whites until they form stiff peaks. Fold into the almond flour mixture. Transfer the mixture to the loaf pan(s) and sprinkle the almonds over the top, if using.

BAKE for 40 to 45 minutes for the large loaf or 30 to 35 minutes for the mini loaves, until golden brown and a toothpick inserted into the center comes out clean.

NUTRITIONAL INFO (PER SERVING)
CALORIES 159, **FAT** 12.6g, **PROTEIN** 3.4g, **CARBS** 2.7g, **FIBER** 0.5g

SOFT SEED BREAD

1½ cups blanched almond flour

¼ cup chia seeds

¼ cup hemp seeds

2 teaspoons psyllium husk

1 teaspoon baking powder

½ teaspoon salt

2 large eggs

4 large egg whites or ½ cup liquid egg whites

4 tablespoons butter, melted

10 drops liquid stevia

MAKES 1 LOAF (12 SERVINGS)

This bread tastes amazing hot or cold. I like to spread it with butter and some sugar-free jelly. You can purchase sugar-free jelly in a variety of flavors at your local grocery store.

PREHEAT the oven to 350°F. Grease a 9- by 5-inch loaf pan.

IN a medium bowl, mix together the almond flour, chia seeds, hemp seeds, psyllium husk, baking powder, and salt.

IN a separate bowl, whisk the eggs and egg whites until frothy. Add the melted butter and stevia and whisk to combine. Add the egg mixture to the almond flour mixture and mix to combine.

POUR into the prepared loaf pan. Bake for 33 to 35 minutes, until golden brown and a toothpick inserted into the center of the bread comes out clean. Serve warm or at room temperature.

TO reheat, place on a microwave-safe plate and heat in the microwave for about 10 seconds.

NUTRITIONAL INFO (PER SERVING)
CALORIES 180, **FAT** 11g, **PROTEIN** 6g, **CARBS** 5.4g, **FIBER** 2.3g

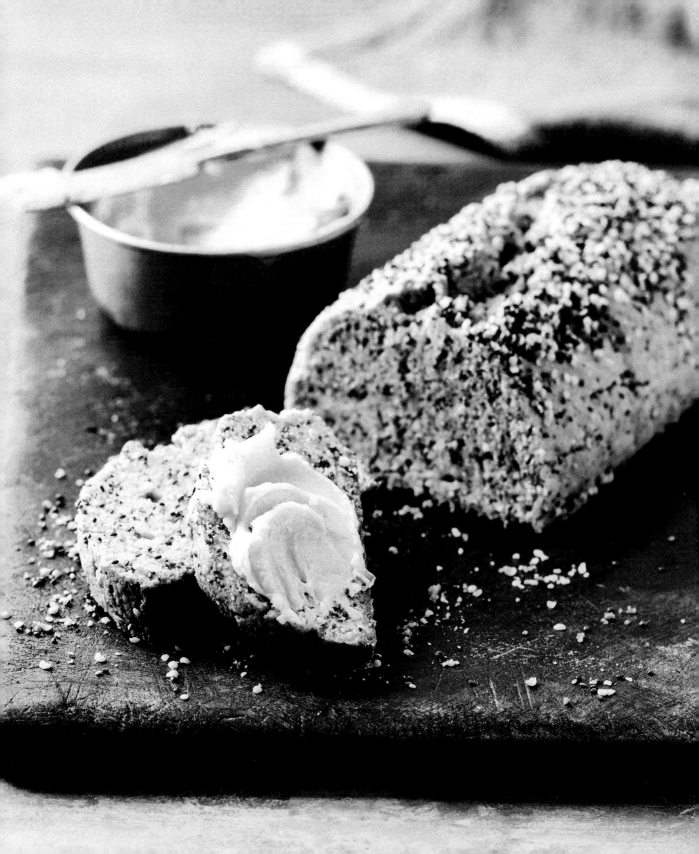

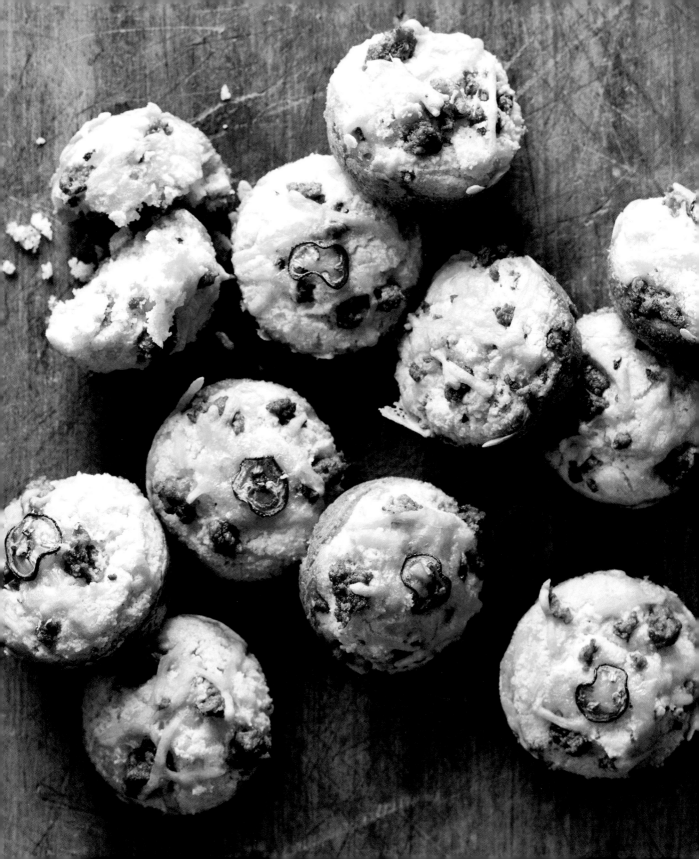

SAUSAGE CHEESE BISCUITS

1 tablespoon extra-virgin
  olive oil

4 ounces pork sausage

2 large eggs

⅓ cup sour cream

4 tablespoons butter, melted

1½ cups blanched almond
  flour

2 teaspoons baking powder

¼ teaspoon garlic powder

¼ teaspoon onion powder

½ teaspoon salt

½ cup shredded cheddar
  cheese, plus more for
  topping

12 jalapeño pepper slices,
  optional

MAKES 12 BISCUITS

If you want a hearty biscuit, this recipe is for you. The biscuits are great served warm or cold. I make them often and never have any left over.

PREHEAT the oven to 350°F. Grease the cups of a 12-cup muffin tin.

IN a medium skillet over medium heat, heat the olive oil. Add the sausage and cook, breaking it up with a wooden spoon, until browned. Drain the fat and set the sausage aside to cool.

IN a medium bowl using a hand mixer, beat the eggs until slightly frothy. Add the sour cream and butter and mix on medium speed until smooth. Add the almond flour, baking powder, garlic powder, onion powder, and salt and mix until fully combined. Add the sausage and mix to combine. Fold in the cheddar cheese.

USE an ice cream scoop to spoon the dough equally into the muffin cups. Top each biscuit with 1 teaspoon shredded cheese and one jalapeño slice, if using. Bake for 24 to 26 minutes, until golden brown and a toothpick inserted into a biscuit comes out clean.

NUTRITIONAL INFO (PER SERVING)
CALORIES 162, **FAT** 9.9g, **PROTEIN** 4.8g, **CARBS** 4g, **FIBER** 0.5g

CORNBREAD CHAFFLES

1 large egg

½ cup plus 2 teaspoons shredded cheddar cheese or part-skim low-moisture mozzarella cheese

5 slices of fresh pickled jalapeño pepper, optional

1 teaspoon Frank's RedHot hot sauce

¼ teaspoon corn flavoring

Pinch salt

MAKES 2 SERVINGS

Corn extract is the secret ingredient that makes these taste just like traditional cornbread. It can be difficult to find cornbread extract at the store, but it's easy to get online. A favorite is OOOFlavors cornbread flavored liquid concentrate.

PREHEAT a mini waffle maker according to the manufacturer's instructions.

IN a small bowl, whisk the egg. Add ½ cup of the cheese, the jalapeño, if using, hot sauce, corn extract, and salt and mix until combined.

ADD 1 teaspoon shredded cheese to the waffle maker and cook for 30 seconds. Add half of the batter and cook for 3 to 4 minutes, until browned and crisp. Repeat with the remaining 1 teaspoon cheese and remaining batter.

NUTRITIONAL INFO (PER SERVING)
CALORIES 150, **FAT** 11.8g, **PROTEIN** 9.6g, **CARBS** 1.1g, **FIBER** 0g

SIMPLE BANANA BREAD

3 large eggs

½ cup extra-virgin olive oil

½ cup coconut milk, cashew milk, or almond milk

1 teaspoon vanilla extract

1 teaspoon banana extract

½ cup monkfruit powdered sweetener

½ cup blanched almond flour

½ cup oat fiber

1 tablespoon unflavored collagen peptides

1 teaspoon xanthan gum

1 teaspoon baking powder

½ teaspoon salt

MAKES 2 MINI LOAVES (10 SERVINGS)

You will be amazed that you can make banana bread without using any bananas. The banana extract stands in for the real thing, which will satisfy your craving without cheating on the diet.

PREHEAT the oven to 350°F. Grease two 6- by 3-inch mini loaf pans.

IN a medium bowl, mix together the eggs, olive oil, coconut milk, vanilla, and banana extract.

IN a separate medium bowl, mix together the sweetener, almond flour, oat fiber, collagen peptides, xanthan gum, baking powder, and salt. Add the flour mixture to the egg mixture and mix to combine.

DIVIDE the mixture between the two prepared loaf pans. Bake for 35 to 38 minutes, until golden brown or a toothpick inserted into the center comes out clean. Serve warm or at room temperature.

NUTRITIONAL INFO (PER SERVING)
CALORIES 197, **FAT** 16g, **PROTEIN** 2.9g, **CARBS** 7.9g, **FIBER** 0.6g

CHEESY GARLIC BREAD CHAFFLES

GARLIC BREAD CHAFFLES

½ cup plus 2 teaspoons shredded part-skim, low-moisture mozzarella cheese

1 large egg

1 teaspoon Italian seasoning

1 teaspoon chive and onion or plain cream cheese

½ teaspoon garlic powder

CHEESY GARLIC BUTTER TOPPING

1 tablespoon butter

½ teaspoon Italian seasoning, plus more for sprinkling

½ teaspoon garlic powder

2 tablespoons shredded part-skim, low-moisture mozzarella cheese

Rao's marinara sauce, warmed, optional

MAKES 2 SERVINGS

I love making keto breads in the mini waffle maker. This recipe adds a cheesy twist to garlic bread and it's to die for. Each waffle is one perfect serving.

FOR THE GARLIC BREAD CHAFFLES

PREHEAT a mini waffle maker according to the manufacturer's instructions. Preheat the oven to 350°F. Line a baking sheet with parchment paper or a silicone mat.

IN a small bowl, mix together ½ cup of the mozzarella, the egg, Italian seasoning, cream cheese, and garlic powder until well combined.

ADD 1 teaspoon shredded cheese to the waffle maker and cook for 30 seconds. Add half of the batter and cook for 4 minutes, or until golden brown. Repeat with the remaining 1 teaspoon cheese and remaining batter. Transfer to the prepared baking sheet.

FOR THE CHEESY GARLIC BUTTER TOPPING

IN a small microwave-safe bowl, heat the butter in the microwave oven until melted, about 10 seconds. Add the Italian seasoning and garlic powder and mix to combine.

BRUSH the topping onto the warm chaffles. Sprinkle the mozzarella and additional Italian seasoning on the chaffles.

BAKE for 5 minutes, or until the cheese is melted. Serve warm with marinara sauce on the side for dipping, if using.

NUTRITIONAL INFO (PER SERVING)
CALORIES 299, **FAT** 9g, **PROTEIN** 48.4g, **CARBS** 6.4g, **FIBER** 2.7g

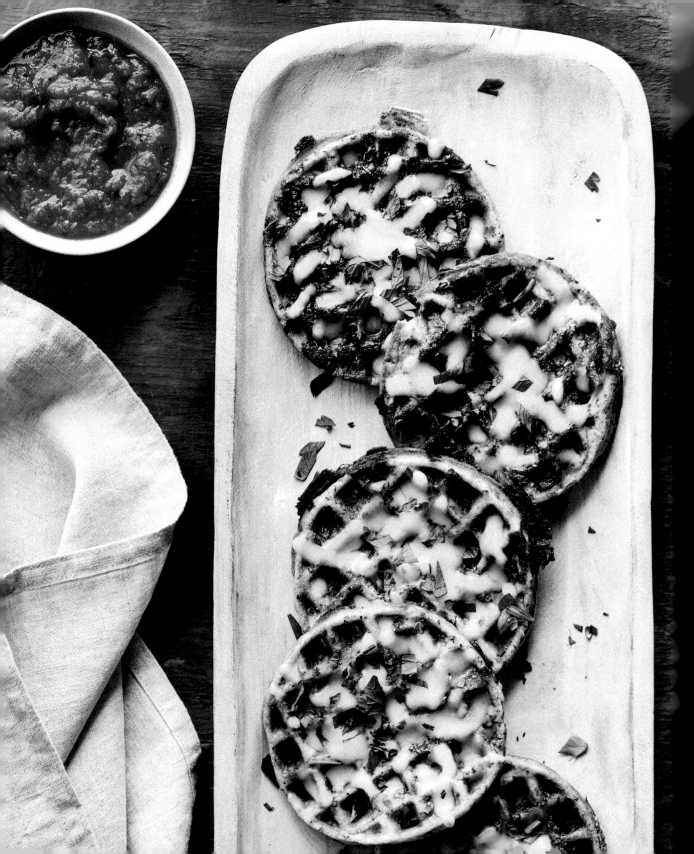

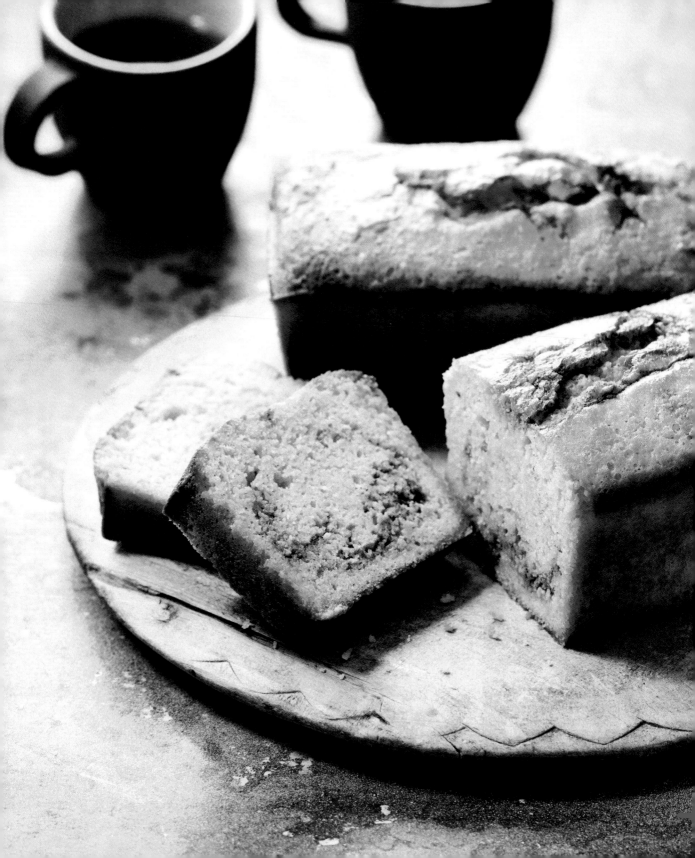

CINNAMON SWIRL BREAD

BREAD

8 ounces cream cheese, at room temperature

8 large eggs, at room temperature

1½ teaspoons vanilla extract

2½ cups blanched almond flour

1½ cups Swerve confectioners' sweetener

8 tablespoons butter

1½ teaspoons baking powder

1 teaspoon unflavored collagen peptides

½ teaspoon salt

CINNAMON SWIRL TOPPING

4 tablespoons butter, melted

¼ cup Swerve brown sugar sweetener

1 teaspoon vanilla extract

¼ teaspoon ground cinnamon

MAKES 2 MINI LOAVES (10 SERVINGS)

The light texture and cinnamon flavor make this bread irresistible. Don't skip the collagen peptides because they give the bread a more traditional texture.

FOR THE BREAD

PREHEAT the oven to 350°F. Grease two 6- by 3-inch mini loaf pans and place on a baking sheet.

IN a small bowl using a hand mixer, beat the cream cheese, eggs, and vanilla until combined. Add the almond flour, confectioners' sweetener, butter, baking powder, collagen peptides, and salt and beat until combined.

DIVIDE the batter between the two prepared loaf pans.

FOR THE CINNAMON SWIRL TOPPING

IN a small bowl, mix together the butter, brown sugar sweetener, vanilla, and cinnamon until combined.

USING a small spoon, spread the topping in a single line along the top of the batter in each pan. Create swirls in the batter by running a butter knife in a criss-cross pattern across the topping.

BAKE for 30 to 35 minutes, until a toothpick inserted into the center of the bread comes out clean. While the bread is warm, remove the loaves from the pans and place on a wire rack to cool.

NUTRITIONAL INFO (PER SERVING)
CALORIES 423, **FAT** 30.4g, **PROTEIN** 10.6g, **CARBS** 8.1g, **FIBER** 1.1g

PUMPKIN BREAD

BREAD

¼ cup pumpkin puree

4 large eggs

2 tablespoons unsweetened almond milk

2 teaspoons vanilla extract

1 cup blanched almond flour

¼ cup oat fiber

¼ cup coconut flour

¼ cup Swerve brown sugar sweetener

¼ cup monkfruit powdered sweetener

1½ teaspoons pumpkin pie spice

1 teaspoon baking powder

GLAZE

2 tablespoons unsweetened almond milk

¾ cup monkfruit powdered sweetener

¼ teaspoon salt

MAKES 2 MINI LOAVES (10 SERVINGS)

I love to make this pumpkin bread around the holidays because the flavors are so festive, plus it makes my kitchen smell really good. The glaze adds just the right amount of sweetness to make the bread a hit. Oat fiber, which should not be confused with oat flour, gives the bread the structure that normally comes from gluten. If you can't find it at the grocery store, it's easy to buy it inexpensively in bulk online.

FOR THE BREAD

PREHEAT the oven to 350°F. Grease two 6- by 3-inch mini bread loaf pans.

IN a large bowl, whisk together the pumpkin, eggs, almond milk, and vanilla until fully combined. Add the almond flour, oat fiber, coconut flour, brown sugar sweetener, powdered sweetener, pumpkin pie spice, and baking powder and mix until fully combined.

DIVIDE the batter between the two prepared pans. Bake for 30 minutes, or until a toothpick inserted into the center comes out clean.

FOR THE GLAZE

IN a small bowl, mix together the almond milk, powdered sweetener, and salt until smooth. Drizzle the glaze over the pumpkin bread, cut into slices, and serve.

NUTRITIONAL INFO (PER SERVING)
CALORIES 127, **FAT** 5.4g, **PROTEIN** 1.8g, **CARBS** 6.4g, **FIBER** 1.7g

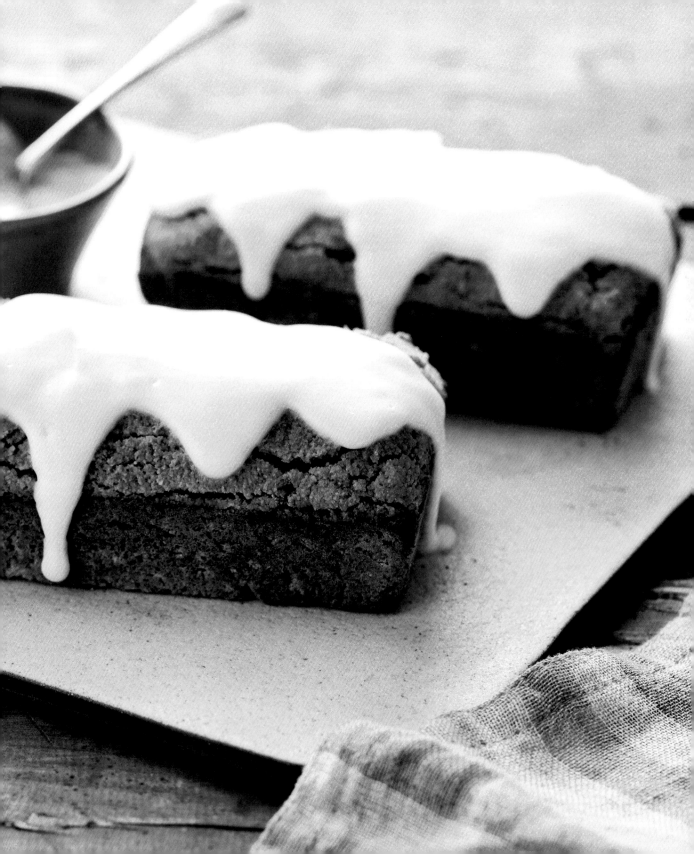

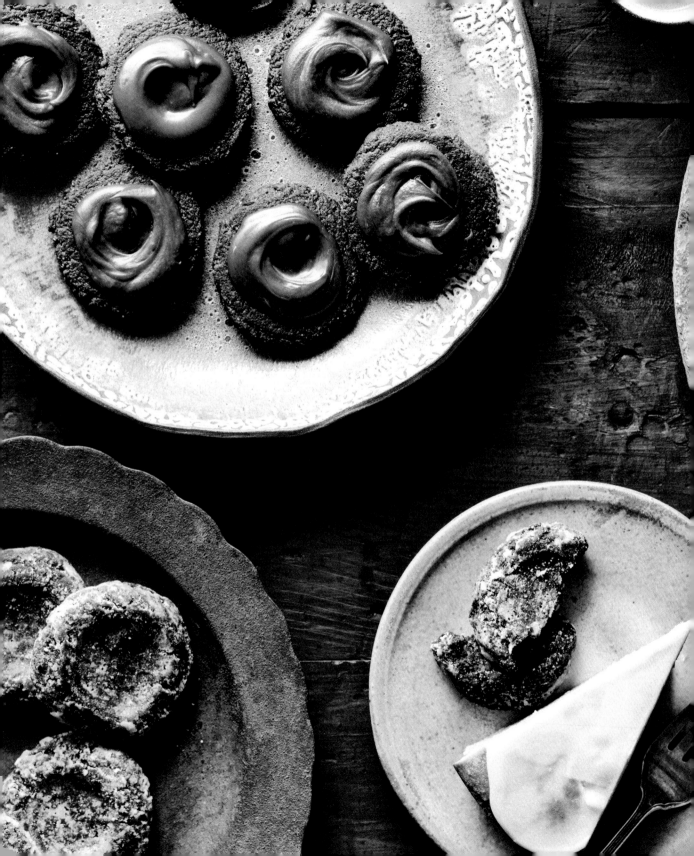

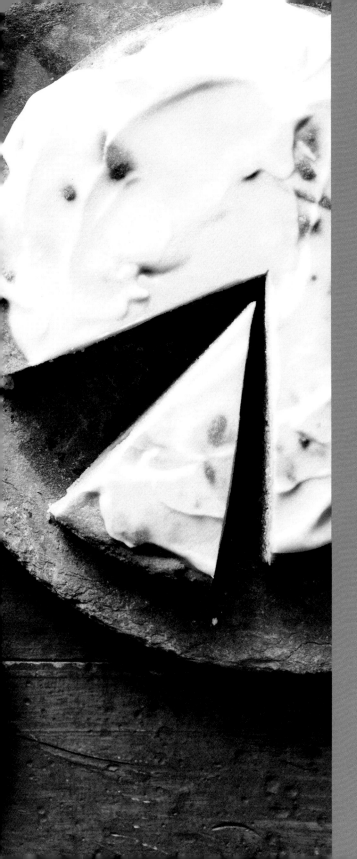

COOKIES & BARS

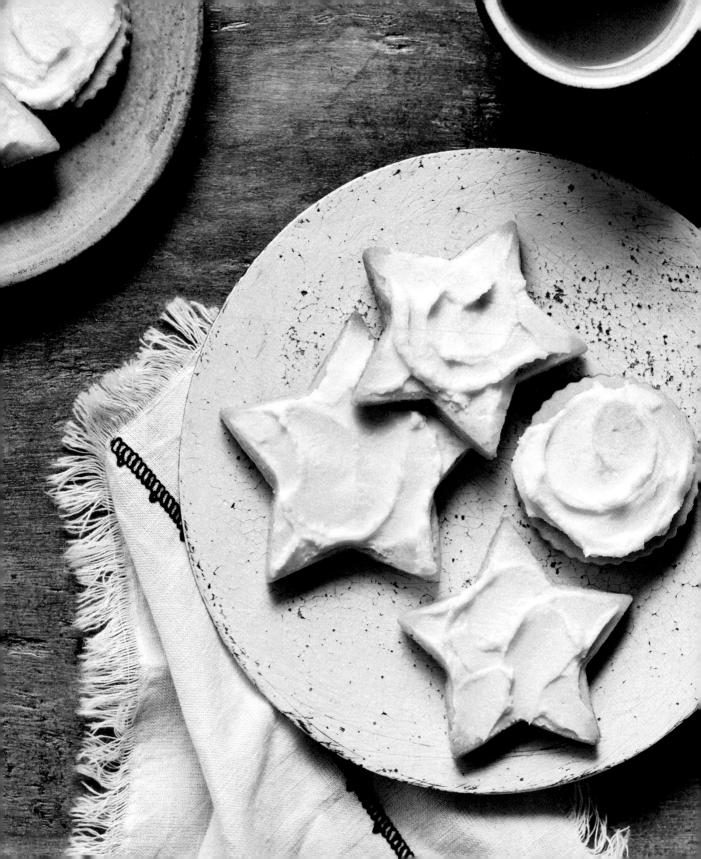

OLD-FASHIONED SUGAR COOKIES

12 tablespoons (1½ sticks) butter

2 ounces cream cheese, at room temperature

1 large egg

1 cup monkfruit powdered sweetener

2 teaspoons vanilla extract

1 teaspoon almond extract

1 teaspoon salt

½ teaspoon liquid stevia

2 cups blanched almond flour

¼ cup coconut flour

2 tablespoons tapioca starch

¼ teaspoon xanthan gum

Buttercream Frosting (page 241)

MAKES 22 LARGE COOKIES

These sugar cookies taste just like Grandma used to make. Get out the cookie cutters and have fun with them. You can cut the carb count by making the cookies much smaller.

IN a large bowl using a hand mixer, beat together the butter and cream cheese until smooth. Add the egg, sweetener, vanilla, almond extract, salt, and stevia and mix well. Add the almond flour, coconut flour, tapioca starch, and xanthan gum and mix well. Cover the bowl with plastic wrap and refrigerate for at least 4 hours, or preferably overnight.

PREHEAT the oven to 350°F. Line baking sheets with parchment paper or silicone mats.

DUST a clean workspace with coconut flour. Using a rolling pin, roll out the dough to ¼ inch thick. Use your favorite cookie cutters to cut shapes of dough and place them ½ inch apart on the prepared baking sheets.

BAKE for 8 to 9 minutes, until lightly browned. Transfer the cookies to a wire rack and let cool for at least 30 minutes to firm up.

SPREAD the buttercream on the cookies and serve.

NUTRITIONAL INFO (PER COOKIE)
CALORIES 170, **FAT** 9.3g, **PROTEIN** 2.2g, **CARBS** 12g, **FIBER** 0.8g

FROSTED VANILLA COOKIES

COOKIES

2 ounces cream cheese, at room temperature

4 tablespoons butter, at room temperature

1 large egg

½ cup Swerve brown sugar sweetener

2 teaspoons vanilla extract

½ teaspoon ground cinnamon

1 cup blanched almond flour

¼ cup coconut flour

½ teaspoon baking powder

½ teaspoon salt

VANILLA FROSTING

3 ounces cream cheese, at room temperature

2 teaspoons monkfruit powdered sweetener

1 teaspoon vanilla extract

Sugar-free sprinkles, optional

MAKES 22 SMALL COOKIES

These cookies don't spread when baking so I press them into shape on the baking sheet before putting them in the oven.

FOR THE COOKIES

PREHEAT the oven to 350°F. Line a baking sheet with parchment paper or a silicone mat.

IN a medium bowl using a hand mixer, beat together the cream cheese and butter until smooth. Add the egg, brown sugar sweetener, vanilla, and cinnamon and mix to combine. Add the almond flour, coconut flour, baking powder, and salt and mix to combine.

USING a cookie scoop, place 22 scoops of dough on the prepared baking sheet. Gently press the cookie dough down slightly to create a flattened round. The cookies will not spread while baking.

BAKE for about 12 minutes, or until lightly browned. Transfer to a wire rack and let cool.

FOR THE FROSTING

IN a small bowl using a hand mixer, beat together the cream cheese, powdered sweetener, and vanilla until smooth. Spread the frosting on the cookies, sprinkle with sugar-free sprinkles, if using, and serve.

NUTRITIONAL INFO (PER COOKIE)
CALORIES 82, **FAT** 5.6g, **PROTEIN** 1.7g, **CARBS** 2.8g, **FIBER** 0.7g

BASIC CHOCOLATE COOKIES

2 large eggs

½ cup almond butter

½ teaspoon liquid stevia

½ teaspoon almond extract

½ teaspoon instant espresso powder

1 cup monkfruit powdered sweetener

½ cup blanched almond flour

⅓ cup unsweetened cocoa powder

1 tablespoon unflavored collagen peptides

¼ teaspoon baking powder

Sugar-Free Ganache (page 240)

MAKES 12 COOKIES

I always bake my chocolate cookies with a small amount of instant espresso powder. This is an old trick that intensifies the chocolate flavor in the most delightful way.

PREHEAT the oven to 350°F. Line a baking sheet with parchment paper or a silicone mat.

IN a medium bowl using a hand mixer, beat the eggs until frothy. Add the almond butter, stevia, almond extract, and espresso powder and beat until smooth. Add the sweetener, almond flour, cocoa powder, collagen peptides, and baking powder and beat until fully combined.

USING a cookie scoop, place 12 scoops of dough on the prepared baking sheet. The dough will be sticky, so use a spoon dipped in water to gently press the cookie dough down slightly to create a flattened round. The cookies will not spread while baking.

BAKE for about 7 minutes, or until slightly firm. They might appear to be slightly undercooked but will be soft and chewy once they have cooled.

SPREAD the cookies with the ganache and serve.

NUTRITIONAL INFO (PER COOKIE)
CALORIES 109, **FAT** 7.7g, **PROTEIN** 4.4g, **CARBS** 4.7g, **FIBER** 2.1g

SOFT SNICKERDOODLES

½ cup allulose sugar

1 teaspoon ground cinnamon

4 ounces cream cheese, at room temperature

4 tablespoons butter, at room temperature

1 large egg

½ cup Swerve brown sugar sweetener

2 teaspoons vanilla extract

½ teaspoon almond extract

1 cup blanched almond flour

¼ cup coconut flour

1 teaspoon xanthan gum

1 tablespoon unsweetened collagen peptides

½ teaspoon baking powder

½ teaspoon salt

MAKES 18 COOKIES

We used allulose sugar as the Snickerdoodle coating because it acts and tastes just like real sugar and, after testing a bunch of other options, found that it's the best for this recipe. The cookies have a wonderful soft and buttery texture.

PREHEAT the oven to 350°F. Line a large baking sheet with parchment paper or a silicone mat.

IN a small bowl, mix together the allulose and cinnamon. Set aside.

IN a medium bowl using a hand mixer, beat together the cream cheese and butter until smooth.

ADD the egg, sweetener, vanilla, and almond extract and mix to combine. Add the almond flour, coconut flour, xanthan gum, collagen peptides, baking powder, and salt and mix to combine.

USE a cookie scoop to portion the dough into 18 pieces. Roll each piece into a ball, roll the ball in the allulose mixture, and place on the prepared baking sheet. Gently press the cookie dough slightly to create to create a flattened round. The cookies will spread during the baking process.

BAKE for about 12 minutes, or until lightly browned. Transfer to a wire rack and let cool.

NUTRITIONAL INFO (PER COOKIE)
CALORIES 96, **FAT** 6.3g, **PROTEIN** 2.6g, **CARBS** 3g, **FIBER** 0.9g

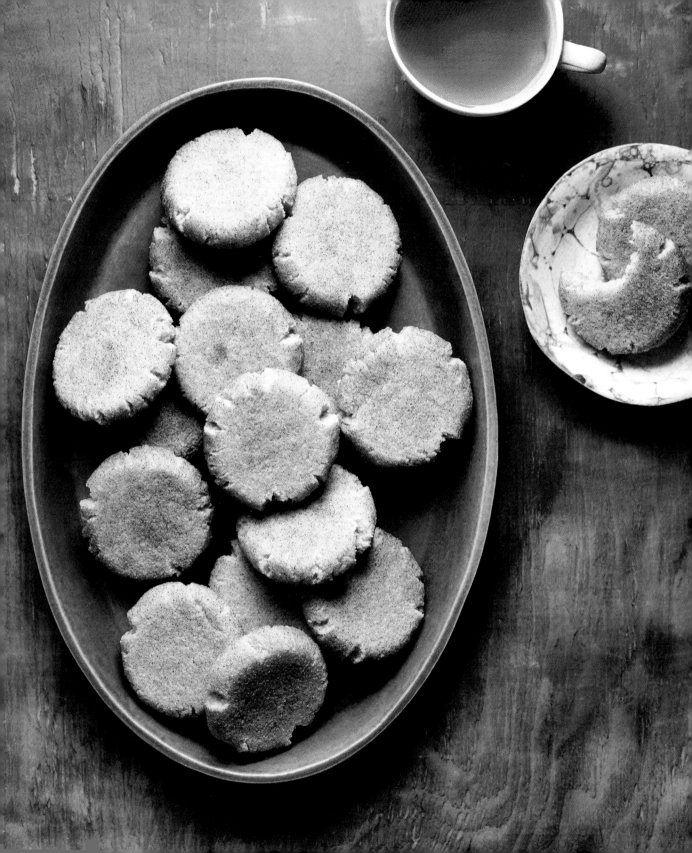

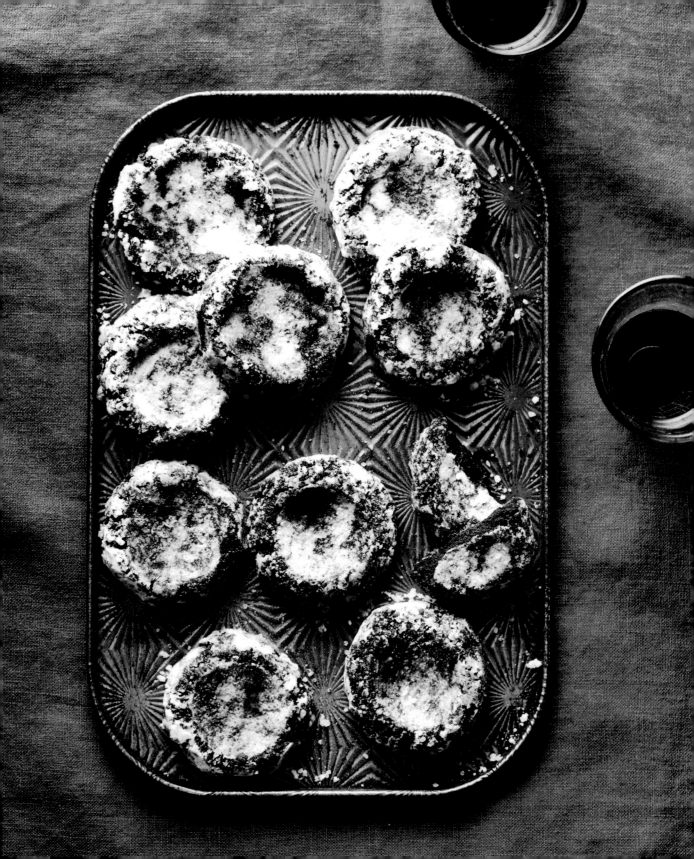

FUDGY CRINKLE COOKIES

COOKIES

2 large eggs

½ cup almond butter

½ teaspoon liquid stevia

½ teaspoon almond extract

½ teaspoon instant espresso powder

½ cup blanched almond flour

⅓ cup unsweetened cocoa powder

1 tablespoon unflavored collagen peptides

1 cup monkfruit powdered sweetener

¼ teaspoon baking powder

CRINKLE COATING

1 tablespoon xylitol

½ cup monkfruit powdered sweetener, plus more for dusting

MAKES 12 COOKIES

The crinkle coating in this recipe uses xylitol and monkfruit powdered sweetener, which together add the perfect level of sweetness along with the beautiful white coating that makes the cookies so special.

FOR THE COOKIES

PREHEAT the oven to 350°F. Line a baking sheet with parchment paper or a silicone mat.

IN a medium bowl using a hand mixer, beat the eggs until frothy. Add the almond butter, stevia, almond extract, and espresso powder and beat until smooth. Add the almond flour, cocoa powder, collagen peptides, monkfruit sweetener, and baking powder and mix until fully combined.

USING a cookie scoop, place 12 scoops of dough on the prepared baking sheet. The dough will be sticky, so use a spoon dipped in water to gently press the cookie dough down slightly to create a flattened round. The cookies will not spread while baking.

FOR THE CRINKLE COATING

IN a small bowl, mix together the xylitol and monkfruit sweetener. Roll each piece of dough in the mixture and return them to the baking sheet.

BAKE for 7 to 10 minutes, or until slightly firm. They might appear to be slightly undercooked but will be soft and chewy once they have cooled. Once cool, dust the cookies with additional monkfruit sweetener and serve.

NUTRITIONAL INFO (PER COOKIE)
CALORIES 108, **FAT** 7.7g, **PROTEIN** 4.3g, **CARBS** 5.2g, **FIBER** 2g

DOUBLE-CHOCOLATE COOKIES WITH GANACHE

COOKIES

2 large eggs

½ cup almond butter

½ teaspoon liquid stevia

½ teaspoon almond extract

½ teaspoon instant espresso powder

1 cup monkfruit powdered sweetener

½ cup blanched almond flour

⅓ cup unsweetened cocoa powder

1 teaspoon xanthan gum

1 tablespoon unflavored collagen peptides

¼ teaspoon baking powder

CHOCOLATE GANACHE

½ cup heavy whipping cream

4 ounces Lily's stevia-sweetened chocolate chips

MAKES 12 COOKIES

If you are a chocolate lover, this recipe is for you! The frosting of ganache gives the cookies an extra indulgent creamy chocolate flavor that will make you very happy. For the ganache, I use Lily's chocolate chips, which are sweetened with stevia. Don't use erythritol in the ganache because the mixture will seize up, preventing it from becoming smooth and creamy.

FOR THE COOKIES

PREHEAT the oven to 350°F. Line a baking sheet with parchment paper or a silicone mat.

IN a medium bowl using a hand mixer, beat the eggs until frothy. Add the almond butter, stevia, almond extract, and espresso powder and beat until smooth. Add the sweetener, almond flour, cocoa powder, xanthan gum, collagen peptides, and baking powder and continue mixing until the ingredients are fully combined.

USING a cookie scoop, place 12 scoops on the prepared baking sheet. The dough will be slightly sticky, so use a spoon dipped in water to spread the dough into a round cookie shape.

BAKE for about 10 to 12 minutes, until slightly firm. They will seem slightly undercooked but will firm up once they have cooled. Transfer to a wire rack and let cool.

FOR THE GANACHE

STOVETOP METHOD: In a small saucepan over medium heat, bring the cream to a simmer; do not let it boil. Remove from the heat, add the chocolate chips, and let sit for 5 to 10 minutes, until the

(continued)

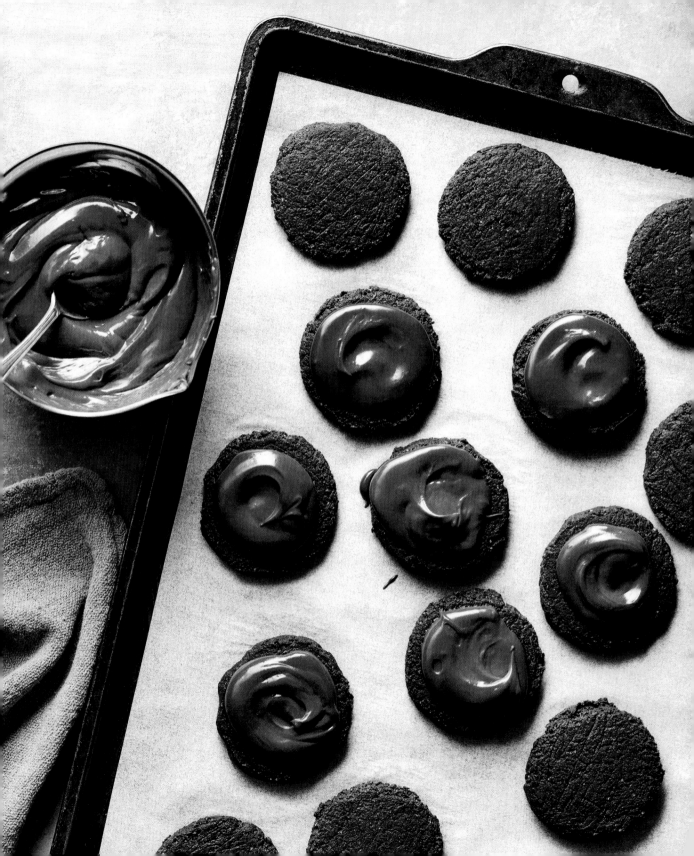

chocolate is melted. Whisk the mixture slowly, gradually increasing speed until the mixture is emulsified and creamy.

MICROWAVE METHOD: In a microwave-safe bowl, add the cream and microwave for 1 minute, or until the cream is between 90°F and 110°F. Add the chocolate chips and cover the bowl with plastic wrap. Let sit for about 2 minutes, until the chocolate is melted. Whisk the mixture until creamy.

LET the ganache cool before spreading onto the cookies.

NUTRITIONAL INFO (PER COOKIE)
CALORIES 125, **FAT** 9.5g, **PROTEIN** 4.5g, **CARBS** 4.9g, **FIBER** 2g

SPICY MEXICAN HOT CHOCOLATE COOKIES

2 large eggs

½ cup almond butter

½ teaspoon liquid stevia

½ teaspoon vanilla extract

½ teaspoon instant espresso powder

1 cup monkfruit powdered sweetener

½ cup blanched almond flour

⅓ cup unsweetened cocoa powder

1 tablespoon unflavored collagen peptides

2 teaspoons ground cinnamon

1 teaspoon chili powder

¼ teaspoon baking powder

⅛ teaspoon cayenne pepper, optional

Sugar-Free Ganache (page 240)

MAKES 12 COOKIES

If you are a fan of Mexican hot chocolate then you will love the bite of spice in this cookie.

PREHEAT the oven to 350°F. Line a baking sheet with parchment paper or a silicone mat.

IN a medium bowl using a hand mixer, beat the eggs until frothy. Add the almond butter, stevia, vanilla, and espresso powder and beat until smooth. Add the sweetener, almond flour, cocoa powder, collagen peptides, cinnamon, chili powder, baking powder, and cayenne, if using, and beat until fully combined.

USING a cookie scoop, place 12 scoops of dough on the prepared baking sheet. The dough will be slightly sticky, so use a spoon dipped in water to spread the dough into a round cookie shape.

BAKE for about 7 minutes, until slightly firm. They will seem slightly undercooked but will be soft and chewy once they have cooled. Transfer to a wire rack and let cool.

SPREAD the ganache on the cookies and serve.

NUTRITIONAL INFO (PER COOKIE)
CALORIES 114, **FAT** 7.8g, **PROTEIN** 5.3g, **CARBS** 5.3g, **FIBER** 2.3g

CHOCOLATE MINT COOKIES

COOKIES

2 large eggs

½ cup almond butter

½ teaspoon liquid stevia

½ teaspoon peppermint extract

1 cup monkfruit powdered sweetener

½ cup blanched almond flour

⅓ cup unsweetened cocoa powder

¼ teaspoon baking powder

1 tablespoon unflavored collagen peptides

CHOCOLATE GANACHE

½ cup heavy whipping cream

4 ounces Lily's stevia-sweetened chocolate chips

½ teaspoon peppermint extract

MAKES 12 COOKIES

Peppermint extract is a key ingredient that adds the peppermint flavor to these delightful cookies so be sure to buy a quality product, either online or at your local grocery store. I also like to use 8 drops of OOOFlavors Girly Cookies mint flavored liquid concentrate. Don't use erythritol to sweeten the ganache because the mixture will seize up, preventing it from becoming smooth and creamy.

FOR THE COOKIES

PREHEAT the oven to 350°F. Line a baking sheet with parchment paper or a silicone mat.

IN a medium bowl using a hand mixer, beat the eggs until frothy. Add the almond butter, stevia, and peppermint extract and mix until smooth. Add the sweetener, almond flour, cocoa powder, baking powder, and collagen peptides and beat until combined.

USING a cookie scoop, place 12 portions of dough on the prepared baking sheet. The dough will be slightly sticky, so use a spoon dipped in water to spread the dough into a round cookie shape.

BAKE for about 7 minutes, or until slightly firm. They will seem slightly undercooked but will be soft and chewy once they have cooled. Transfer to a wire rack and let cool.

FOR THE GANACHE

STOVETOP METHOD: In a small saucepan over medium heat, bring the cream to a simmer; do not let it boil. Remove from the heat, add the chocolate chips, and let sit for 5 to 10 minutes, until the chocolate is melted. Add the peppermint extract and whisk the mixture slowly, gradually increasing speed until the mixture is emulsified and creamy.

MICROWAVE METHOD: In a microwave-safe bowl, add the cream and microwave for 1 minute, or until the cream is between 90°F and 110°F. Add the chocolate chips and cover the bowl with plastic wrap. Let sit for about 2 minutes, until the chocolate is melted. Add the peppermint extract and whisk the mixture until creamy.

LET the ganache cool before spreading onto the cookies.

NUTRITIONAL INFO (PER COOKIE)
CALORIES 129, **FAT** 9.5g, **PROTEIN** 5.4g, **CARBS** 4.9g, **FIBER** 2g

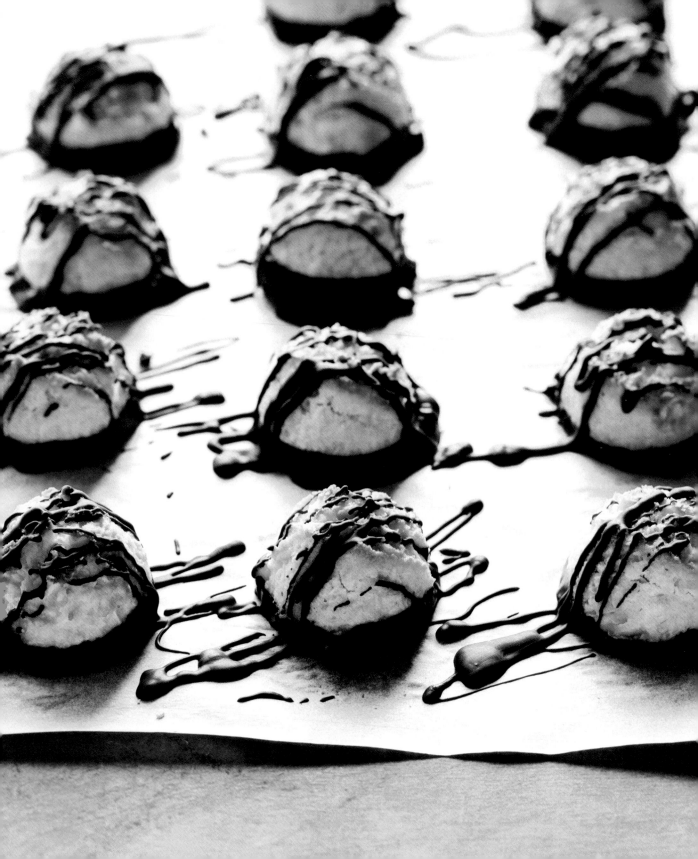

COCONUT-CHOCOLATE MACAROONS

5 large egg whites

¾ cup monkfruit powdered
sweetener

½ cup blanched almond flour

1 teaspoon vanilla extract

½ teaspoon salt

2½ cups unsweetened
coconut flakes

½ cup Lily's stevia-
sweetened dark chocolate
chips

1 teaspoon coconut oil

MAKES 18 MACAROONS

This recipe is a coconut and chocolate lover's dream. It's one of
my favorite flavor combinations.

PREHEAT the oven to 350°F. Line a baking sheet with parchment
paper or a silicone mat. Have a sheet of parchment paper ready.

IN a medium bowl, mix together the egg whites, sweetener,
almond flour, vanilla, and salt. Add the coconut flakes and mix until
completely combined.

FORM 1 tablespoon of the mixture into a ball and place on the baking
sheet. Repeat with the rest of the mixture to make 18 macaroons.

BAKE for 15 minutes, or until the coconut is lightly browned.
Transfer to a wire rack and let cool.

IN a small microwave-safe bowl, mix together the chocolate
chips and coconut oil and heat in the microwave oven for about
10 seconds. Stir and continue to heat in 10-second intervals at
50 percent power until the chocolate chips have melted.

DIP the bottoms of the macaroons in the melted chocolate and
place them on the sheet of parchment paper. Drizzle the remaining
chocolate over the tops of the macaroons.

NUTRITIONAL INFO (PER MACAROON)
CALORIES 134, **FAT** 10.4g, **PROTEIN** 3.2g, **CARBS** 6g, **FIBER** 1.9g

PEPPERMINT MERINGUE KISSES

½ cup egg whites

½ teaspoon cream of tartar

10 drops liquid monkfruit sweetener, plus more if desired

1 teaspoon clear vanilla extract

3 drops peppermint extract

No-taste red food coloring

MAKES 45 MINI KISSES (9 SERVINGS)

These pretty kisses are perfect for parties as they display beautifully. You will need a piping bag or a large zip-top bag to make the meringues. Be sure to use a no-taste red food coloring because regular red adds a bitter taste. Clear vanilla extract will ensure that each kiss is a bright, snowy white.

PREHEAT the oven to 200°F. Line a baking sheet with parchment paper or a silicone mat.

IN a medium bowl using a hand mixer, beat the egg whites and cream of tartar on medium-low for 2 to 3 minutes, until frothy. Increase the speed to medium and slowly beat in the liquid sweetener. Increase the speed to high, add the vanilla and peppermint extract, and continue to beat until stiff peaks form.

DIP the point of a skewer into the food coloring. Starting from the inside tip of the piping bag or bottom corner of a zip-top bag, draw a line of food coloring up the bag. Repeat this step four or five times, until you have drawn lines of food coloring around the entire bag.

USING a large spatula, transfer the egg white mixture into the bag and close the bag with a clip or by twisting the end. Cut off about 1 inch of the tip of the piping bag or the corner of the zip-top bag. Pipe about 45 kisses onto baking sheet. They can be piped close together because they will not spread while baking.

BAKE for about 15 minutes, just enough to dry them out. They should not brown.

STORE the kisses in a covered container at room temperature for up to 2 weeks.

NUTRITIONAL INFO (PER 5 MINI KISSES)
CALORIES 8, **FAT** 0g, **PROTEIN** 1.3g, **CARBS** 0.3g, **FIBER** 0g

CHOCOLATE CHAFFLE COOKIES

CHAFFLES

1 large egg

2 tablespoons cream cheese, at room temperature

1 tablespoon unsweetened black cocoa

1 tablespoon monkfruit powdered sweetener

1 tablespoon mayonnaise

1 teaspoon vanilla extract

¼ teaspoon baking powder

¼ teaspoon instant espresso powder

Pinch salt

FROSTING

4 tablespoons monkfruit powdered sweetener

4 tablespoons cream cheese, at room temperature

½ teaspoon vanilla extract

MAKES 3 CHAFFLES (6 SERVINGS)

This recipe tastes almost just like an Oreo cookie because of the black cocoa, which gives it a smooth chocolate flavor, and the espresso powder, which intensifies the flavor of the chocolate. The black cocoa also gives the cookie that very dark brown color we all know and love. The mayonnaise adds extra moisture and balance to the cookie.

FOR THE CHAFFLES

PREHEAT a mini waffle maker according to the manufacturer's instructions.

IN a small bowl, whisk the egg. Add the cream cheese, black cocoa, sweetener, mayonnaise, vanilla, baking powder, espresso powder, and salt and whisk until smooth.

POUR one-third of the batter into the mini waffle maker and cook for 2½ to 3 minutes, until fully cooked. Repeat with the rest of the batter to make three chaffles. Transfer to a wire rack and let cool.

FOR THE FROSTING

IN a small bowl, mix together the sweetener, cream cheese, and vanilla until smooth.

CUT each chaffle in half, spread with frosting, and serve.

NUTRITIONAL INFO (PER ½ CHAFFLE)
CALORIES 69, **FAT** 5g, **PROTEIN** 3.5g, **CARBS** 2.7g, **FIBER** 0.7g

LEMON-KISS GLAZED COOKIES

COOKIES

4 tablespoons butter, at room temperature

2 ounces cream cheese, at room temperature

1 large egg

½ cup Swerve brown sugar sweetener

2 teaspoons vanilla extract

½ teaspoon lemon extract

1 cup blanched almond flour

¼ cup coconut flour

1 tablespoon unflavored collagen peptides

½ teaspoon baking powder

½ teaspoon salt

LEMON GLAZE

3 tablespoons monkfruit powdered sweetener

2 tablespoons lemon juice

Sugar-free sprinkles, optional

Lemon zest, optional

MAKES 20 COOKIES

Lemon lovers rejoice, as we now have a fantastic lemon cookie that's keto friendly.

FOR THE COOKIES

PREHEAT the oven to 350°F. Line a baking sheet with parchment paper or a silicone mat.

IN a medium bowl using a hand mixer, beat together the butter and cream cheese. Add the egg, brown sugar sweetener, vanilla, and lemon extract and beat to combine. Add the almond flour, coconut flour, collagen peptides, baking powder, and salt and beat to combine.

USE a cookie scoop to portion the dough into 20 pieces, roll them into balls, and place on the prepared baking sheet. Gently press each ball slightly to create a flattened round. These cookies will not spread while baking.

BAKE for 12 minutes, or until lightly browned. Transfer to a wire rack and let cool.

FOR THE LEMON GLAZE

IN a small bowl, mix together the powdered sweetener, lemon juice, and 1 tablespoon of water until smooth. Drizzle the glaze over the cookies, sprinkle with sugar-free sprinkles and lemon zest, if you like, and serve.

NUTRITIONAL INFO (PER COOKIE)
CALORIES 91, **FAT** 6.1g, **PROTEIN** 2.4g, **CARBS** 3g, **FIBER** 0.7g

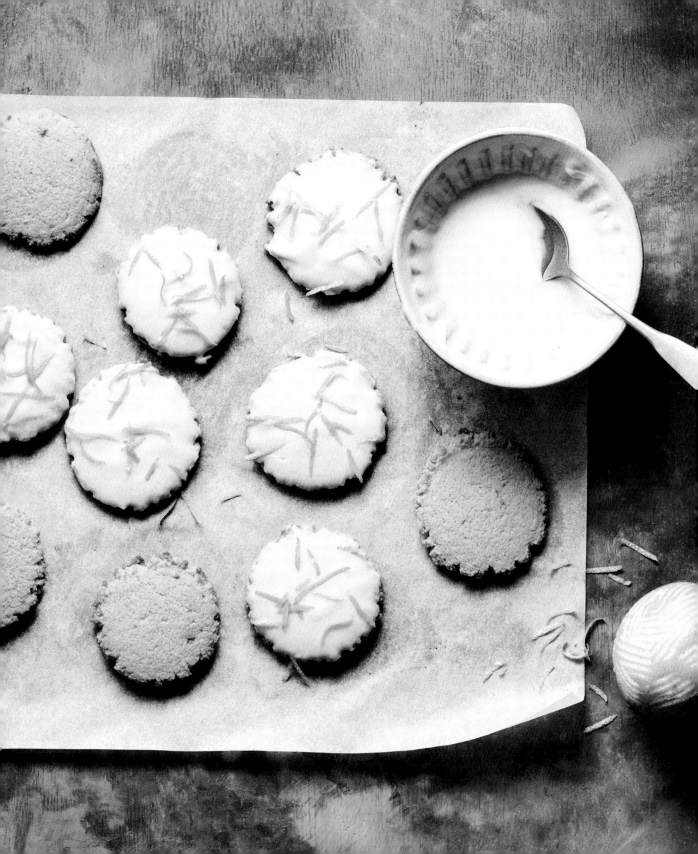

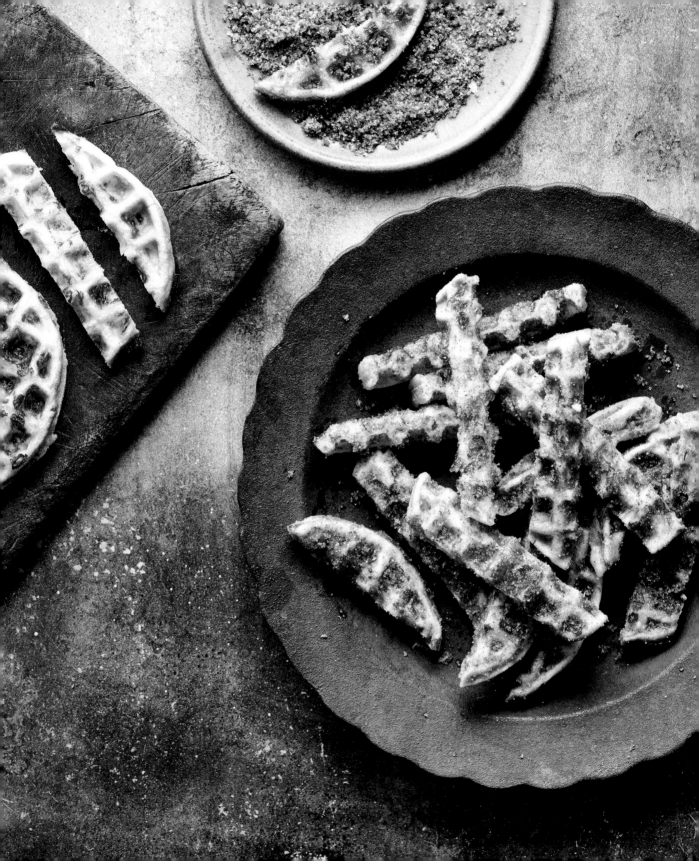

CHAFFLE CHURROS

2 tablespoons Swerve brown sugar sweetener

½ teaspoon ground cinnamon

1 large egg

½ cup shredded part-skim, low-moisture mozzarella cheese

MAKES 2 SERVINGS

If you are in the mood for something sweet, these chaffle churros hit the spot. The warm chaffle soaks up the cinnamon sugar perfectly, and when I eat them it's hard to believe they are keto friendly. I'm sure glad they are!

IN a small bowl, mix together the sweetener and cinnamon. Set aside.

PREHEAT a mini waffle maker according to the manufacturer's instructions.

IN a small bowl, whisk the egg. Add the mozzarella cheese and mix to combine.

POUR half of the batter into the mini waffle maker and cook for about 4 minutes, until golden brown. Repeat with the remaining batter.

WHILE the chaffles are still hot, cut each one into five slices and dredge in the cinnamon mixture. Serve warm.

NUTRITIONAL INFO (PER SERVING)
CALORIES 77, **FAT** 2.4g, **PROTEIN** 12.1g, **CARBS** 5.7g, **FIBER** 0.9g

FROSTED SUGAR-COOKIE BARS

8 tablespoons (1 stick) cold butter

2 ounces cream cheese, at room temperature

1 large egg

½ cup monkfruit powdered sweetener

2 teaspoons vanilla extract

1 cup blanched almond flour

¼ cup coconut flour

½ teaspoon baking powder

½ teaspoon salt

Buttercream Frosting (page 241)

MAKES 8 BARS

I use a loaf pan to make eight perfectly sized bars. If you like, you can use a little red food coloring to make the frosting pink and then top them with sugar-free sprinkles. I like the Good Dee's brand of sugar-free sprinkles, which are pretty and taste good.

PREHEAT the oven to 350°F. Grease a 9- by 5-inch loaf pan.

IN a small bowl using a hand mixer, beat the butter and cream cheese until smooth. Add the egg, sweetener, and vanilla and beat until combined. Add the almond flour, coconut flour, baking powder, and salt until smooth.

POUR the batter into the prepared loaf pan and smooth the top. Bake for 18 to 20 minutes, until a toothpick inserted into the center comes out clean. Transfer to a wire rack to cool completely.

SPREAD the frosting over the cookie bars. Cut into eight bars and serve.

NUTRITIONAL INFO (PER BAR)
CALORIES 234, **FAT** 17.4g, **PROTEIN** 4.1g, **CARBS** 5.9g, **FIBER** 1.8g

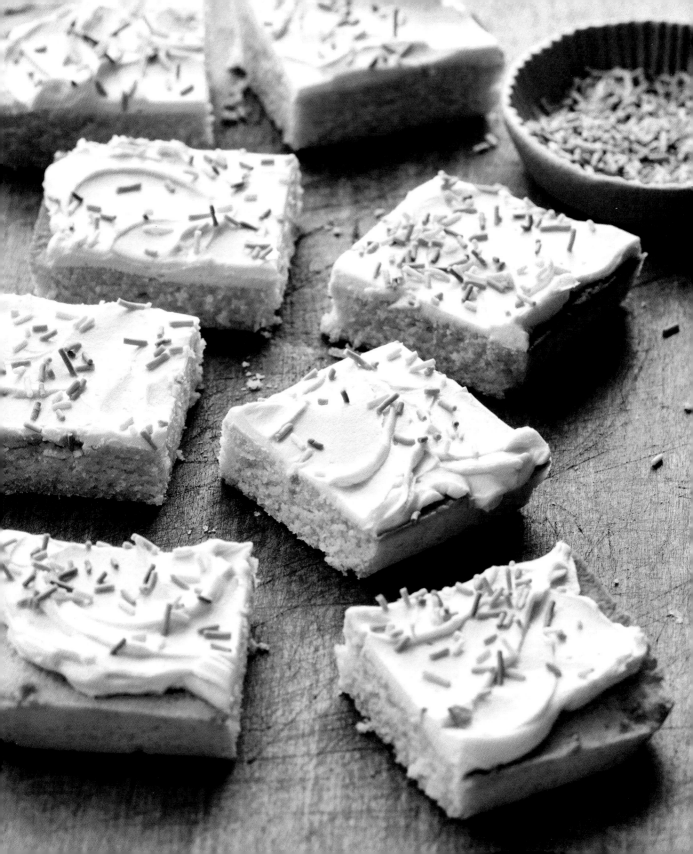

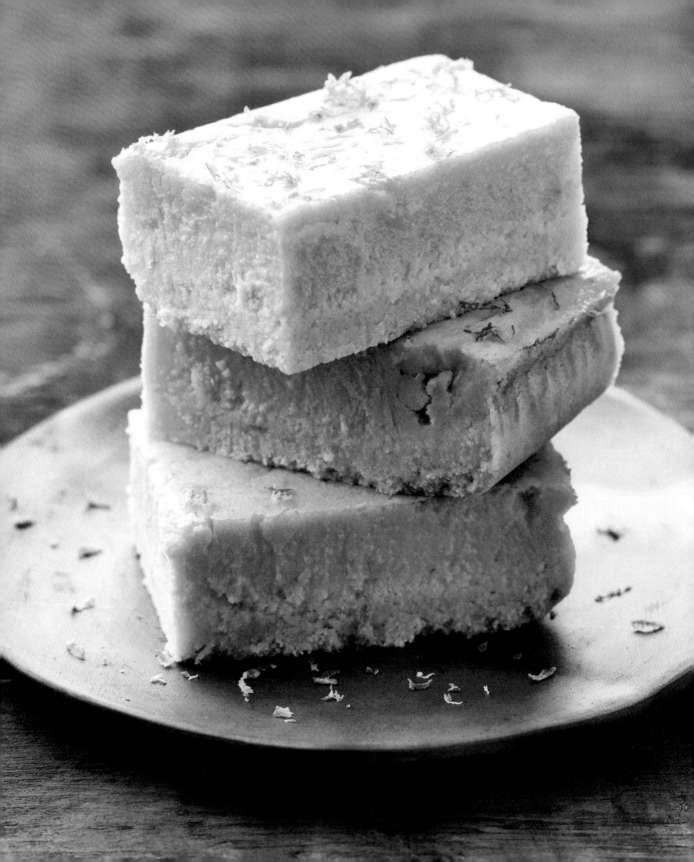

KEY LIME BARS

CRUST

4 tablespoons cold butter

2 large eggs

1 cup blanched almond flour

¾ cup monkfruit granulated sweetener

⅓ cup coconut flour

1 tablespoon vanilla extract

½ teaspoon salt

FILLING

8 large eggs

2 large egg yolks

1 cup key lime juice

1 cup monkfruit powdered sweetener

3 tablespoons coconut flour

Grated zest of 1 lime

MAKES 12 BARS

These bars have a fantastic key lime filling with a cookie crust. I often make the bars for parties or potluck gatherings.

FOR THE CRUST

PREHEAT the oven to 365°F. Grease a 9-inch square baking pan.

IN a medium bowl using a hand mixer, beat the butter and eggs with a hand mixer until they come together. Add the almond flour, monkfruit sweetener, coconut flour, vanilla, and salt and beat until fully combined. Spread the mixture in the prepared baking pan. Set aside.

FOR THE FILLING

IN a medium bowl using a hand mixer, beat the eggs, egg yolks, lime juice, powdered sweetener, coconut flour, and lime zest and beat until smooth.

POUR the filling over the crust mixture and spread evenly. Bake for 30 to 35 minutes, until fully cooked in the middle. The edges will be browned and the top will be dry. Cut into 12 bars and serve.

NUTRITIONAL INFO (PER BAR)
CALORIES 174, **FAT** 10g, **PROTEIN** 7.7g, **CARBS** 7.6g, **FIBER** 2.2g

FUDGY BROWNIES

2 large eggs

½ cup extra-virgin olive oil

¼ cup canned pure
   pumpkin puree

2 tablespoons unsweetened
   sunflower butter

1 teaspoon vanilla extract

¼ teaspoon liquid stevia

¾ cup unsweetened cocoa
   powder

¾ cup monkfruit powdered
   sweetener

1 tablespoon Swerve brown
   sugar sweetener

½ teaspoon espresso powder

½ teaspoon salt

⅛ teaspoon ground
   cinnamon

MAKES 12 BARS

I tested numerous versions of this recipe in my quest to find the perfect brownie texture and taste—and I think I finally succeeded. The brownies are rich, fudgy, and tender. In a word? Delightful!

PREHEAT the oven to 365°F. Line a 9-inch square baking pan with parchment or a silicone mat.

IN a large bowl using a hand mixer, beat the eggs, olive oil, pumpkin puree, sunflower butter, vanilla, and stevia until fully combined, about 2 minutes. Add the cocoa, powdered sweetener, brown sugar sweetener, espresso powder, salt, and cinnamon and beat until combined.

SPREAD the mixture evenly in the prepared baking pan. Bake for 15 minutes, or until the batter is set and not jiggly. Transfer the baking pan to a wire rack and let cool slightly before cutting into 12 bars and serving.

NUTRITIONAL INFO (PER BAR)
CALORIES 134, **FAT** 12.1g, **PROTEIN** 2.6g, **CARBS** 5.3g, **FIBER** 1.6g

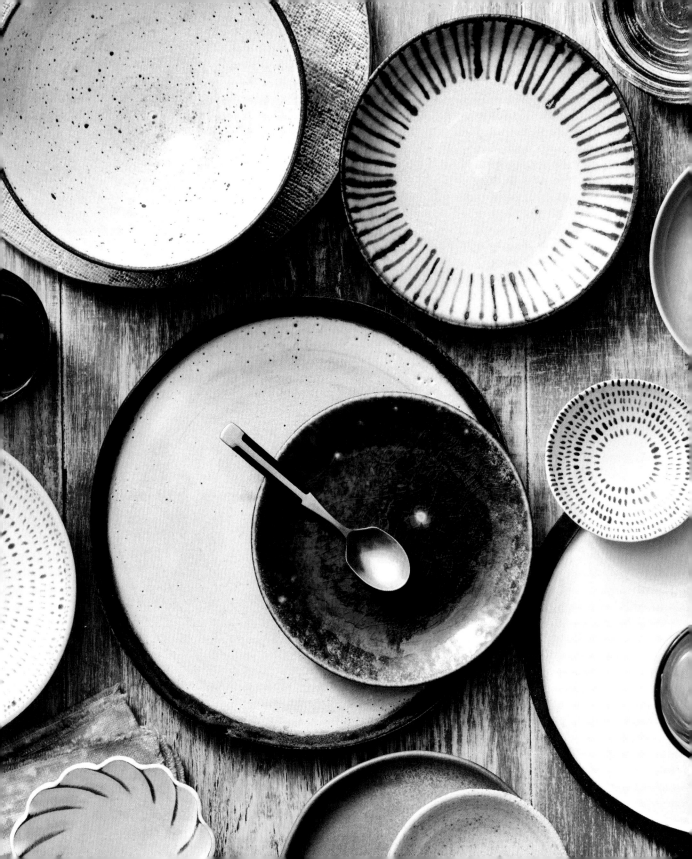

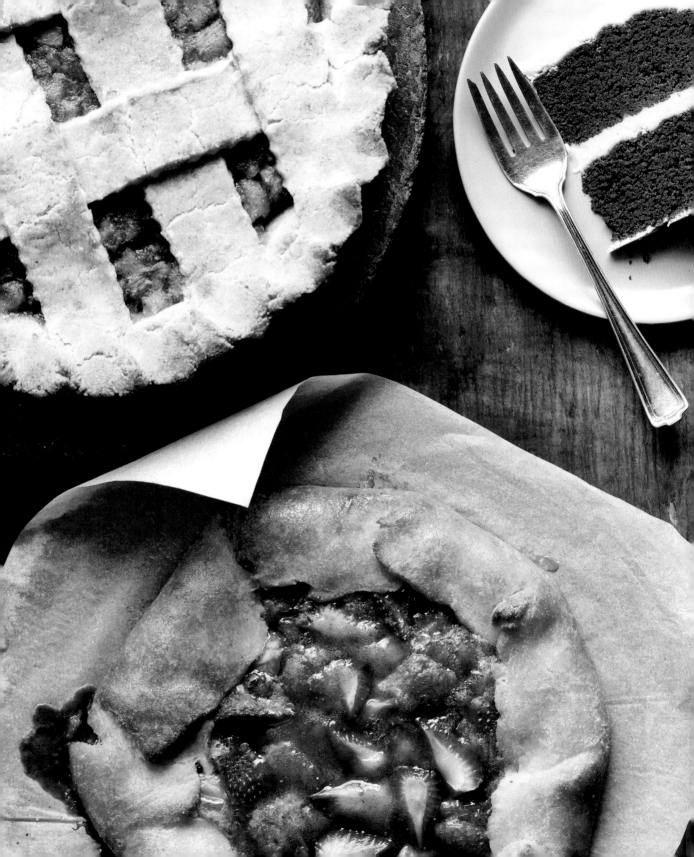

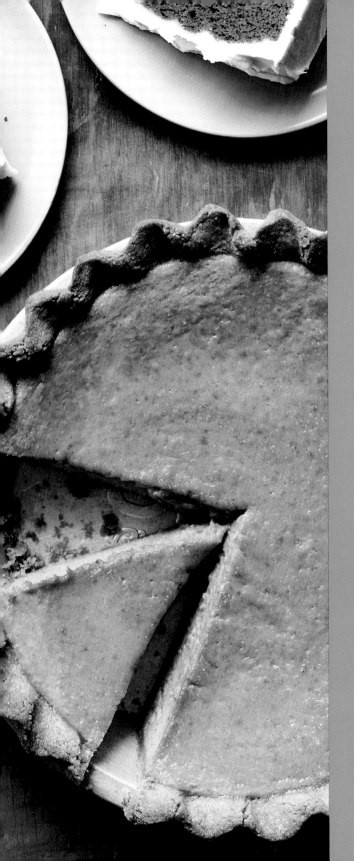

CAKES & PIES

GLAZED CINNAMON COFFEE CAKE

CAKE

3 large eggs

1 teaspoon vanilla extract

½ cup blanched almond flour

½ cup oat fiber

½ cup erythritol or Swerve granulated sweetener

½ cup monkfruit sweetener

1 tablespoon unflavored collagen peptides

1½ teaspoons baking powder

1 teaspoon xanthan gum

1 teaspoon ground cinnamon

½ teaspoon salt

GLAZE

4 tablespoons butter

¼ cup erythritol or Swerve confectioners' sweetener

½ cup heavy whipping cream

1 teaspoon vanilla extract

½ teaspoon ground cinnamon

MAKES 8 SERVINGS

Make this cake to enjoy alongside a hot cup of coffee or tea.

FOR THE CAKE

PREHEAT the oven to 350°F. Grease a 9-inch round cake pan.

IN a medium bowl, mix together the eggs and vanilla until frothy.

IN a separate bowl, mix together the almond flour, oat fiber, erythritol, monkfruit sweetener, collagen peptides, baking powder, xanthan gum, cinnamon, and salt. Add the almond flour mixture to the egg mixture and mix until well combined.

TRANSFER the batter to the prepared cake pan. Bake for 35 to 38 minutes, until golden brown on top or a toothpick inserted in the center comes out clean. Transfer to a wire rack to cool.

FOR THE GLAZE

IN a medium saucepan over medium heat, melt the butter. Add the erythritol and cook, stirring frequently, until fully dissolved. Add the cream, vanilla, and cinnamon and cook, stirring, for about 5 minutes. Remove the pan from the heat.

PLACE the cake on a serving plate and brush with the glaze. Serve warm or cold.

NUTRITIONAL INFO (PER SERVING)
CALORIES 156, **FAT** 11.5g, **PROTEIN** 5g, **CARBS** 4.2g, **FIBER** 1g

CINNAMON CHAYOTE UPSIDE-DOWN MINI CAKES

CAKE

8 large eggs, at room temperature

8 ounces cream cheese, at room temperature

2 teaspoons vanilla extract

2½ cups blanched almond flour

1½ cups Swerve granulated sweetener

1 tablespoon unflavored collagen peptides

1½ teaspoons baking powder

1 teaspoon ground cinnamon

½ teaspoon salt

1½ cups Chayote Compote (page 280)

CARAMEL SAUCE

8 tablespoons (1 stick) butter

1½ cups Swerve brown sugar sweetener

2 teaspoons salt

¼ cup heavy whipping cream

¼ teaspoon xanthan gum

1 teaspoon vegetable glycerin, optional

MAKES 8 (4-INCH) MINI BUNDT CAKES (16 SERVINGS)

The chayote compote in this recipe tastes just like hot cinnamon apples! Once you try chayote squash, it will become one of your favorite vegetables. It's a good source of vitamin C, vitamin B_6, folate, dietary fiber, and potassium. Every part of the squash is edible and, although it can be eaten raw and is sometimes shredded to put into salads and slaws, it's more often cooked, like in this recipe.

FOR THE CAKE

PREHEAT the oven to 350°F. Grease eight (4-inch) mini Bundt pans.

IN a small bowl using a hand mixer, beat the eggs, cream cheese, and vanilla until combined. Add the almond flour, granulated sweetener, collagen peptides, baking powder, cinnamon, and salt and beat until combined.

SPOON 3 tablespoons of chayote compote into the bottom of each mini Bundt pan. Spoon the batter over the compote, filling them three-fourths full. Place the Bundt pans on a baking sheet and bake for 30 to 35 minutes, until a toothpick inserted into the center of the cake comes out clean. Unmold the mini cakes, transfer to a wire rack, and let cool

FOR THE CARAMEL SAUCE

IN a medium saucepan, over medium-high heat, melt and heat the butter, stirring frequently, until browned, 2 to 3 minutes. Add the brown sugar sweetener and salt and cook, whisking, until the sweetener has fully dissolved and the mixture starts to bubble. Reduce the heat to low, add the cream and xanthan gum, and cook, stirring, until the mixture thickens slightly. Remove from the heat. The sauce will thicken as it cools.

(continued)

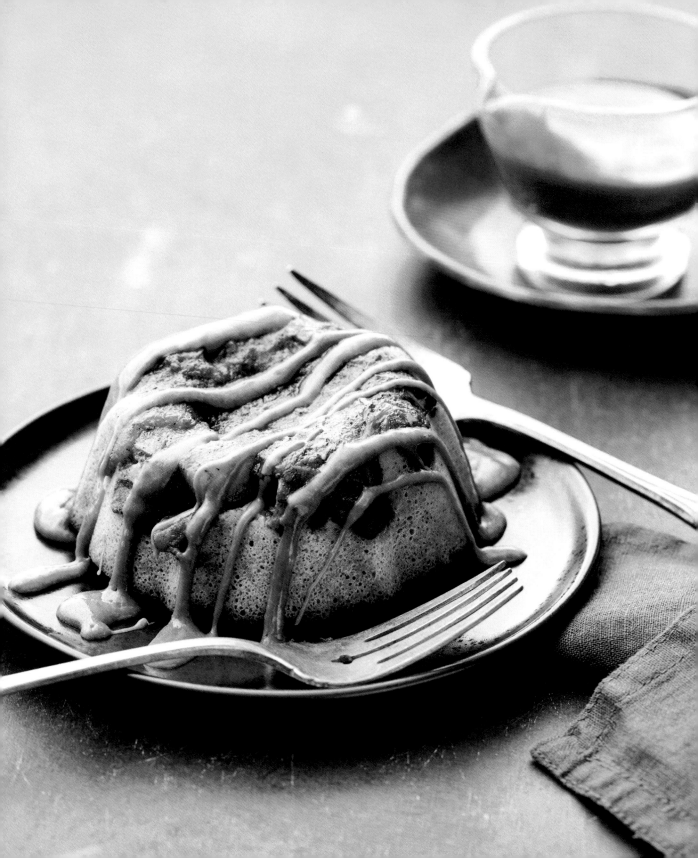

IF using, add the vegetable glycerin to prevent the sauce from crystalizing. I think it creates a smooth texture that makes it worth using.

CUT a mini cake in half, place on a plate, and drizzle with caramel sauce just before serving.

NUTRITIONAL INFO (PER SERVING)
CALORIES 202, **FAT** 13.7g, **PROTEIN** 5.9g, **CARBS** 5.4g, **FIBER** 0.8g

BANANA CAKE

CAKE

3 large eggs

½ cup extra-virgin olive oil

¼ cup coconut milk, cashew milk, or almond milk

1 teaspoon vanilla extract

1 teaspoon banana extract

½ cup Swerve confectioners' sweetener

½ cup blanched almond flour

½ cup oat fiber

2 tablespoons unflavored collagen peptides

1 teaspoon xanthan gum

1 teaspoon baking powder

½ teaspoon salt

GLAZE

½ cup Swerve confectioners' sweetener

1 teaspoon vanilla extract

MAKES 20 SERVINGS

Bananas have been off the menu since I started keto. That's why I'm super impressed with LorAnn Banana Bakery Emulsion: It makes this cake taste like real bananas. So, you can have your cake and eat it too!

FOR THE CAKE

PREHEAT the oven to 350°F. Grease a 9-inch round cake pan.

IN a medium bowl using a hand mixer, beat the eggs, oil, coconut milk, vanilla, and banana extract until smooth.

IN a separate medium bowl, mix together the sweetener, almond flour, oat fiber, collagen peptides, xanthan gum, baking powder, and salt. Add the flour mixture to the egg mixture and mix until combined.

POUR the batter into the prepared cake pan. Bake for 28 to 30 minutes, until golden brown or a toothpick inserted into the center of the cake comes out clean. Transfer the pan to a wire rack.

FOR THE GLAZE

IN a small bowl, mix together the sweetener, vanilla, and 2 teaspoons water until smooth. Spread the glaze over the hot cake and serve.

NUTRITIONAL INFO (PER SERVING)
CALORIES 87, **FAT** 7.4g, **PROTEIN** 2.5g, **CARBS** 8.3g, **FIBER** 0.3g

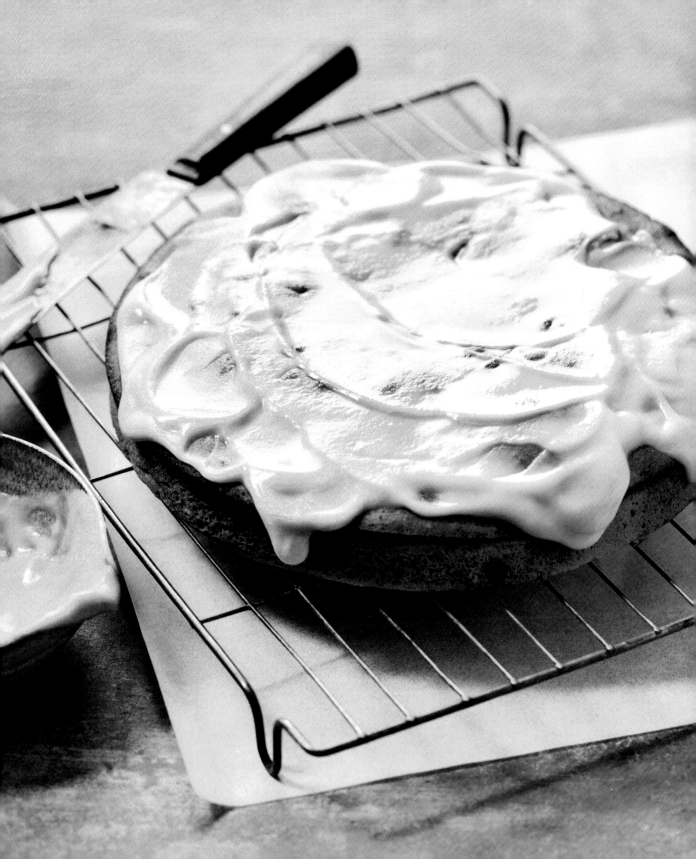

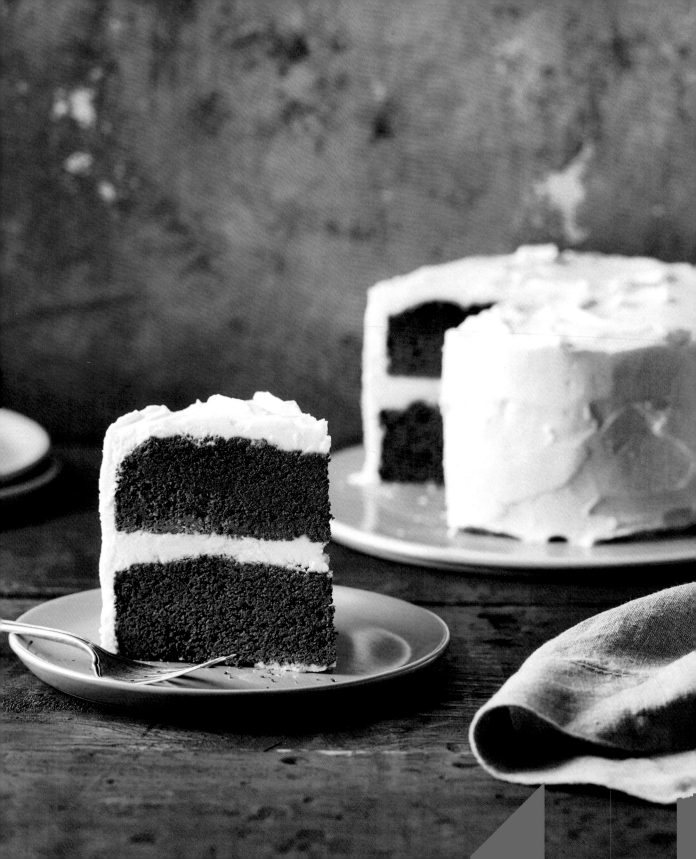

RED VELVET CAKE

CAKE

4 large eggs

1 cup Pyure organic granulated stevia

8 tablespoons (1 stick) butter, melted

¼ cup heavy whipping cream

2 tablespoons MCT oil

1 teaspoon vanilla extract

1 teaspoon AmeriColor super red food coloring

1 cup blanched almond flour

½ cup coconut flour

2 tablespoons unsweetened Dutch-processed cocoa powder

1 teaspoon baking powder

½ teaspoon pink Himalayan salt

½ teaspoon guar gum

½ teaspoon baking soda

FROSTING

12 ounces cream cheese, at room temperature

¾ cup heavy whipping cream

½ cup Pyure organic granulated stevia

2 teaspoons clear vanilla extract

MAKES 8 SERVINGS

I use Dutch-processed cocoa powder and AmeriColor super red food coloring to perfect this gorgeous cake. If you decide to omit the food coloring, that's fine, the cake will still taste wonderful.

FOR THE CAKE

PREHEAT the oven to 350°F. Grease two 6-inch round cake pans.

IN a large bowl using a hand mixer, beat the eggs, granulated stevia, butter, cream, MCT oil, vanilla, and food coloring until smooth. Add the almond flour, coconut flour, cocoa powder, baking powder, salt, guar gum, and baking soda and beat to combine.

DIVIDE the batter equally between the two cake pans. Bake for 30 minutes, until a toothpick inserted into the centers of the cakes comes out clean.

REMOVE the cakes from the pans, transfer to a wire rack, and let cool.

FOR THE FROSTING

IN a bowl using a hand mixer, beat the cream cheese, cream, granulated stevia, and vanilla until smooth.

TO frost the cake, place the first cake layer on a serving platter and frost the top of the cake. Place the second layer on top of the first layer, frost the sides of the cake, and finish by frosting the top of the cake.

NUTRITIONAL INFO (PER SERVING)
CALORIES 459, **FAT** 38g, **PROTEIN** 9.4g, **CARBS** 10g, **FIBER** 3.2g

LEMON CHAFFLE CAKE

CHAFFLES

2 ounces cream cheese, at room temperature

2 large eggs

2 tablespoons coconut flour

2 teaspoons butter, melted

1 teaspoon monkfruit powdered sweetener

1 teaspoon baking powder

½ teaspoon lemon extract

20 drops LorAnn cake batter flavoring

FROSTING

½ cup heavy whipping cream

1 tablespoon monkfruit powdered sweetener

¼ teaspoon lemon extract

½ teaspoon grated lemon zest, optional

MAKES 4 SERVINGS

This is a really good dessert that can be made quickly in a mini waffle maker. The chaffle tastes like traditional cake and has a beautiful lemon flavor. The frosting adds the perfect finishing touch. The chaffles are stacked with frosting layered in between, making this a tall impressive mini cake. I love using an ice cream scoop to scoop the batter because it holds about 3 tablespoons, which fits perfectly in the mini waffle maker.

FOR THE CHAFFLE

PREHEAT a mini waffle maker according to the manufacturer's instructions.

IN a blender, combine the cream cheese, eggs, coconut flour, melted butter, sweetener, baking powder, lemon extract, and cake batter flavoring and blend until smooth, about 2 minutes.

WITH an ice cream scoop, fill the waffle iron with one full scoop of batter. Cook for 4 minutes, or until the chaffle is golden brown. Transfer to a wire rack and let cool. Repeat with the rest of the batter to make four chaffles.

FOR THE FROSTING

IN a medium bowl using a hand mixer, beat the cream, sweetener, lemon extract, and lemon zest, if using, until stiff peaks form.

TO assemble the cake, place one chaffle on a small serving plate. Spread frosting over the chaffle and top with a second chaffle. Spread frosting on the second chaffle and top with the third. Spread another layer of frosting and top with the last chaffle. Spread frosting on the top chaffle. Cut into six slices and serve.

NUTRITIONAL INFO (PER SERVING)
CALORIES 171, **FAT** 15g, **PROTEIN** 5.2g, **CARBS** 6g, **FIBER** 1.3g

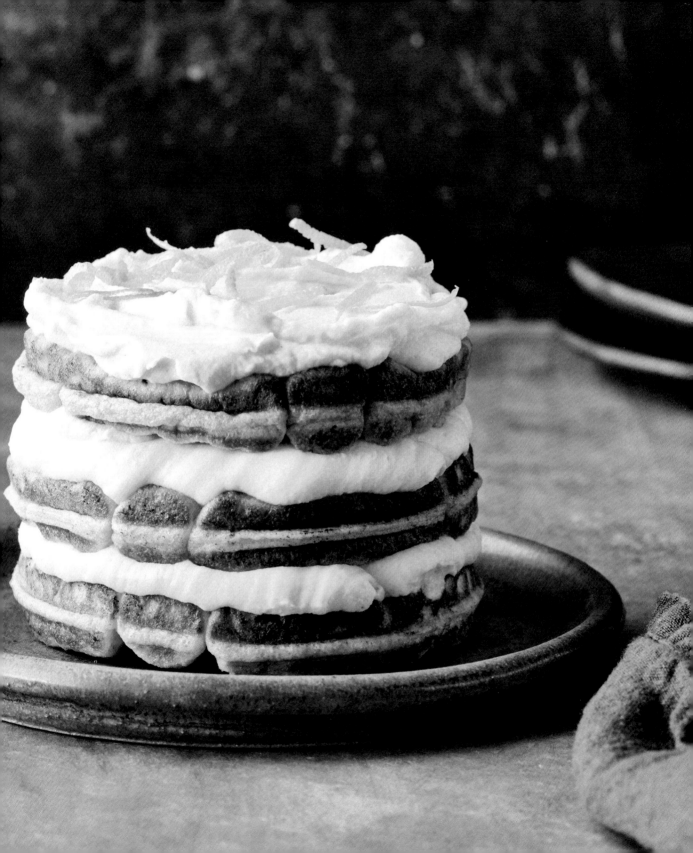

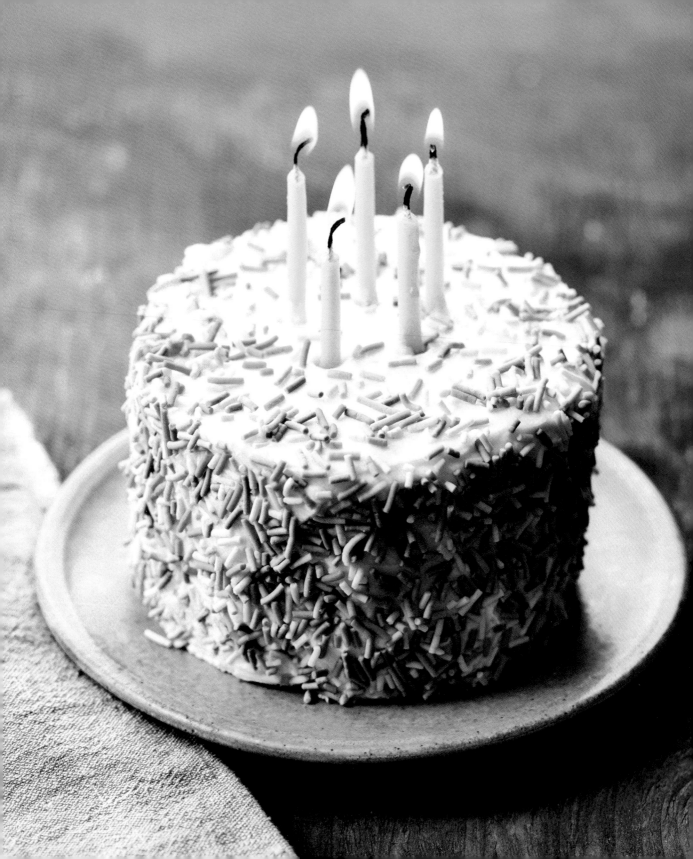

BIRTHDAY CHAFFLE CAKE

CHAFFLES

2 large eggs

¼ cup blanched almond flour

2 tablespoons butter, melted

2 tablespoons cream cheese, at room temperature

2 tablespoons Swerve confectioners' sweetener

1 teaspoon coconut flour

1 teaspoon LorAnn cake batter flavoring

½ teaspoon vanilla extract

½ teaspoon baking powder

¼ teaspoon xanthan gum

VANILLA WHIPPED CREAM

½ cup heavy whipping cream

2 tablespoons Swerve confectioners' sweetener

½ teaspoon vanilla extract

Sugar-free sprinkles, optional

MAKES 6 SERVINGS

This is the recipe I make every year for my birthday. It's a light and fluffy cake with a very airy whipped cream topping. I always stack the chaffles to make a tall cake with layers of whipped cream in between. It's nice to be able to indulge yourself on your birthday without guilt.

FOR THE CHAFFLES

PREHEAT a mini waffle maker according to the manufacturer's instructions.

IN a blender, combine the eggs, almond flour, melted butter, cream cheese, sweetener, coconut flour, cake batter flavoring, vanilla, baking powder, and xanthan gum and blend until smooth and creamy.

WITH an ice cream scoop, fill the waffle iron with one full scoop of batter. Cook for 3 to 4 minutes, until the chaffle is golden brown. Transfer to a wire rack and let cool. Repeat with the rest of the batter to make four chaffles.

FOR THE VANILLA WHIPPED CREAM

IN a bowl using a hand mixer, beat the cream, sweetener, and vanilla until soft peaks form.

TO assemble the cake, place one chaffle on a small serving plate. Spread whipped cream over the chaffle and top with a second chaffle. Spread whipped cream on the second chaffle and top with the third. Spread another layer of whipped cream and top with the last chaffle. Spread whipped cream on the top chaffle, covering the sides if you wish. If desired, top with sugar-free sprinkles. Cut into six slices and serve.

NUTRITIONAL INFO (PER SERVING)
CALORIES 170, **FAT** 13g, **PROTEIN** 2.9g, **CARBS** 8g, **FIBER** 0.4g

ITALIAN CREAM CHAFFLE CAKE

CHAFFLES

4 large eggs

4 ounces cream cheese, at room temperature

¼ cup coconut flour

1 tablespoon butter, melted

1 tablespoon monkfruit sweetener

1 tablespoon blanched almond flour

1½ teaspoons baking powder

1 teaspoon vanilla extract

½ teaspoon ground cinnamon

1 tablespoon shredded unsweetened coconut, plus more for garnish

1 tablespoon chopped walnuts, plus more for garnish

ITALIAN CREAM FROSTING

2 ounces cream cheese, at room temperature

2 tablespoons butter, at room temperature

2 tablespoons monkfruit powdered sweetener

½ teaspoon vanilla extract

MAKES 8 SERVINGS

Although I call for walnuts in the cake, I have also put them on top of the frosting, with very tasty results. You can't go wrong with either choice. You can use a regular size waffle maker for this recipe: Use the batter to make four larger chaffles and stack them to make one impressive cake.

FOR THE CHAFFLES

PREHEAT a mini waffle maker according to the manufacturer's instructions.

IN a blender, mix together the eggs, cream cheese, coconut flour, butter, monkfruit sweetener, almond flour, baking powder, vanilla, and cinnamon and blend until smooth. Add the coconut and walnuts and mix to combine.

WITH an ice cream scoop, fill the waffle iron with one full scoop of batter. Cook for 3 to 4 minutes, until the chaffle is golden brown. Transfer to a wire rack and let cool. Repeat with the rest of the batter to make eight chaffles.

FOR THE ITALIAN CREAM FROSTING

IN a small bowl using a hand mixer, beat the cream cheese, butter, powdered sweetener, and vanilla until smooth.

TO assemble the cake, place one chaffle on a small serving plate. Spread frosting over the chaffle and top with a second chaffle. Spread frosting on the second chaffle and top with the third. Spread another layer of frosting and top with the last chaffle. Spread frosting on the top chaffle. Repeat with the remaining four chaffles and frosting to make two cakes. Top with more walnuts and coconut.

NUTRITIONAL INFO (PER SERVING)
CALORIES 127, **FAT** 9.7g, **PROTEIN** 5.3g, **CARBS** 5.5g, **FIBER** 1.3g

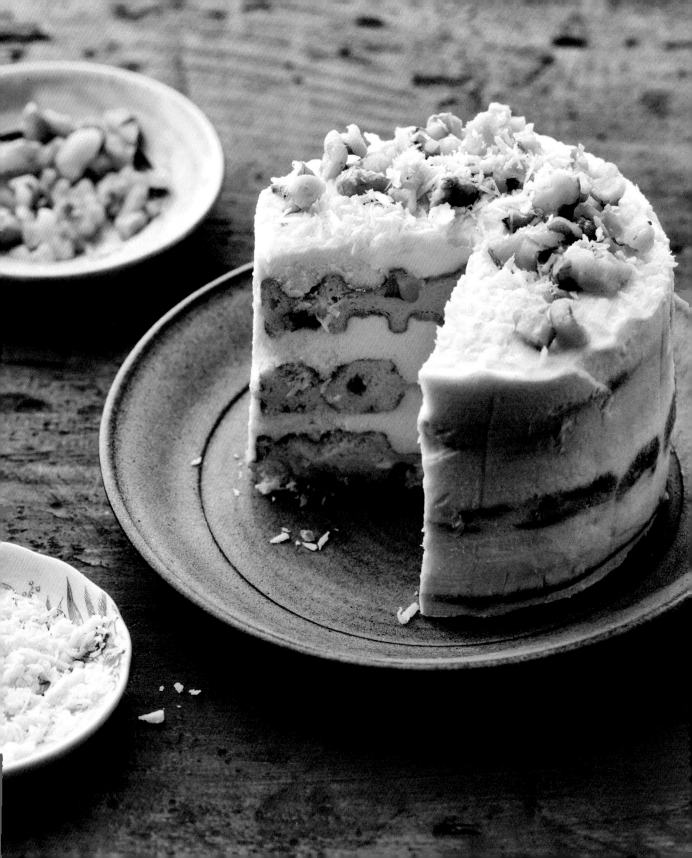

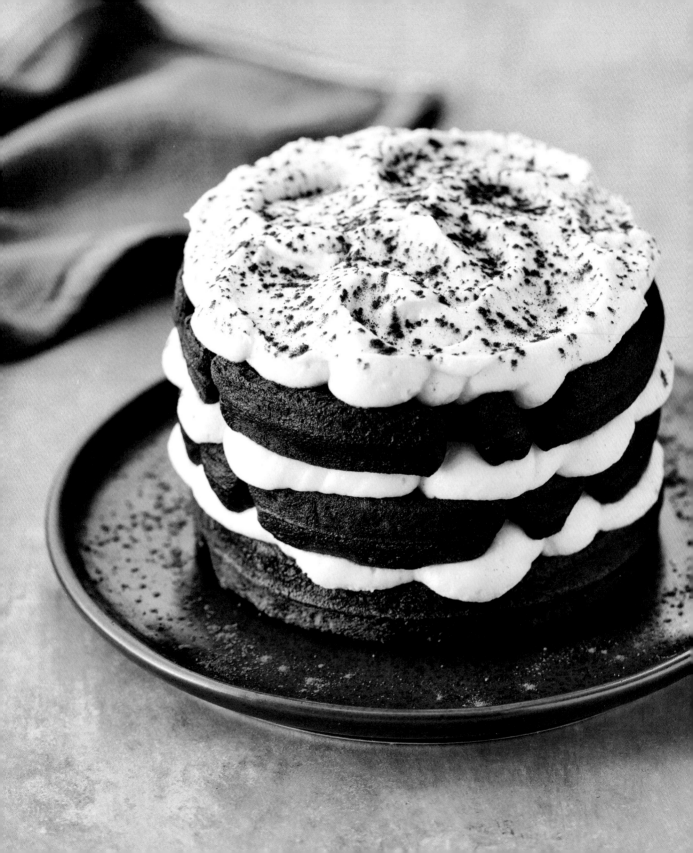

CHOCOLATE WAFFLE CAKE

CHOCOLATE WAFFLES

1 large egg

2 tablespoons unsweetened cocoa powder

2 tablespoons monkfruit powdered sweetener

¼ teaspoon baking powder

FROSTING

¼ cup monkfruit powdered sweetener

¼ cup cream cheese, at room temperature

½ teaspoon clear vanilla extract

MAKES 4 SERVINGS

This chocolate cake is absolutely adorable when served on a mini cake stand. It's a great choice when you need to make a special cake at the last minute.

FOR THE CHOCOLATE WAFFLES

PREHEAT a mini waffle maker according to the manufacturer's instructions.

IN a small bowl, whisk the egg. Add the cocoa, sweetener, and baking powder and mix until smooth.

POUR one-third of the batter in the waffle maker and cook for 2½ to 3 minutes, until fully cooked. Repeat with the rest of the batter to make three waffles. Transfer to a wire rack and cool completely.

FOR THE FROSTING

IN a small bowl using a hand mixer, beat the sweetener, cream cheese, and vanilla until smooth.

TO assemble the cake, place one waffle on a small serving plate. Spread frosting over the waffle and top with a second waffle. Spread frosting on the second waffle. Spread another layer of frosting and top with the last waffle. Spread frosting on the top waffle. Cut into three slices and serve.

NUTRITIONAL INFO (PER SERVING)
CALORIES 90, **FAT** 7.9g, **PROTEIN** 3.1g, **CARBS** 6.9g, **FIBER** 1g

PUMPKIN PIE

½ cup sour cream

4 large eggs, beaten

1 (15-ounce) can pure pumpkin puree

¾ cup Swerve confectioners' sweetener

½ cup heavy whipping cream

1 teaspoon ground cinnamon

½ teaspoon ground ginger

½ teaspoon salt

¼ teaspoon cloves

1 unbaked Flaky Pie Shell (page 243)

MAKES 12 SERVINGS

My family really enjoys this pie during the holidays and it's nice to be able to serve a traditional recipe that doesn't break the keto diet. Top it with sugar-free whipped cream or your favorite keto ice cream.

PREHEAT the oven to 375°F.

IN a large bowl, mix together the sour cream, eggs, pumpkin puree, sweetener, cream, cinnamon, ginger, salt, and cloves and mix until smooth.

POUR the mixture into the unbaked pie crust. Bake for 45 to 50 minutes, until the crust is golden brown and the middle is only slightly jiggly. If the crust edge browns too early, place aluminum foil over the edge to prevent burning.

NUTRITIONAL INFO (PER SERVING)
CALORIES 228, **FAT** 12.1g, **PROTEIN** 4.9g, **CARBS** 9.5g, **FIBER** 1.7g

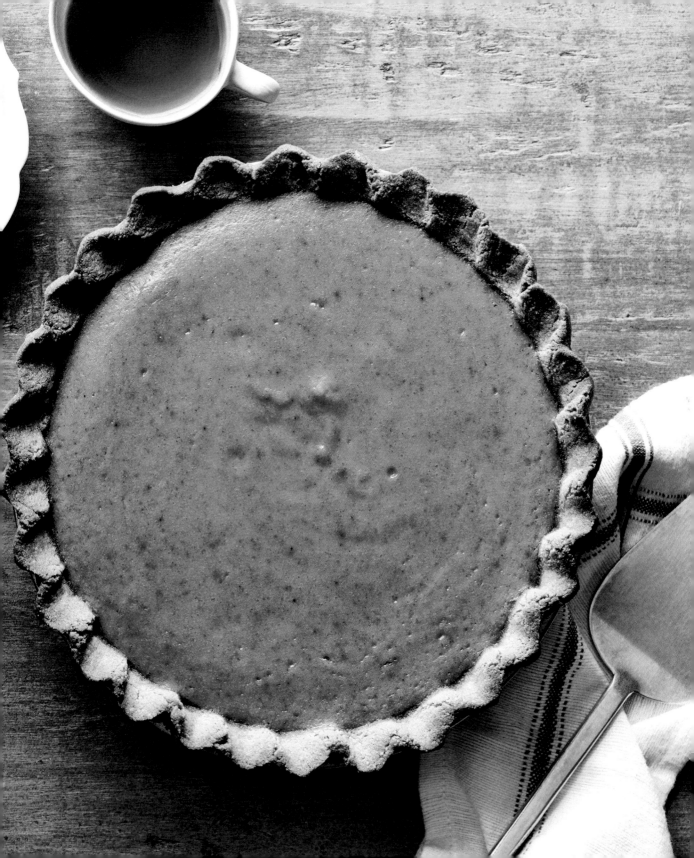

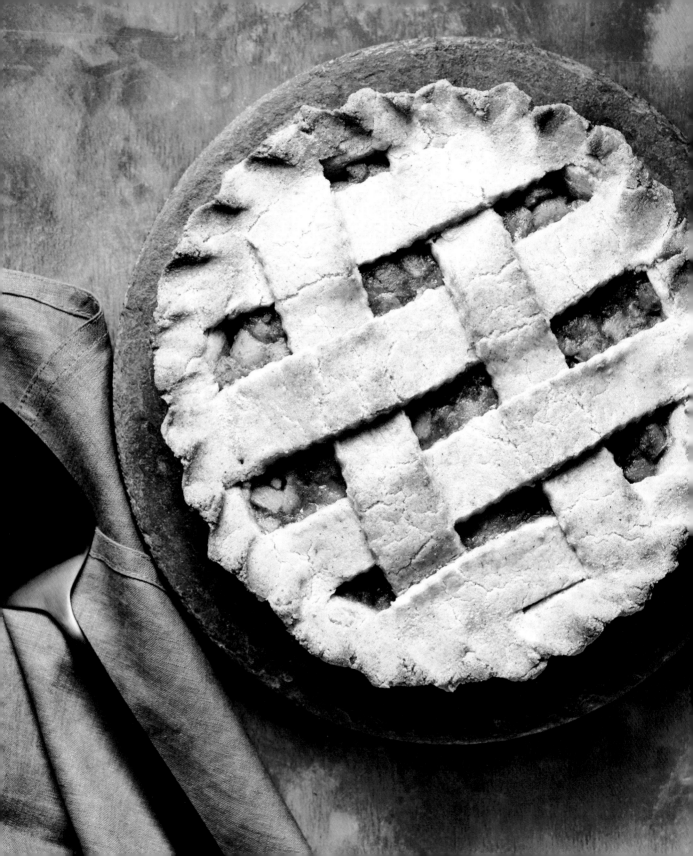

CHAYOTE "APPLE" PIE

12 tablespoons (1½ sticks) butter

2 ounces cream cheese

2 large eggs

1 teaspoon salt

2 cups blanched almond flour

¼ cup coconut flour

2 tablespoons psyllium husk

2 tablespoons tapioca starch

¼ teaspoon xanthan gum

Chayote Compote (page 280)

MAKES 12 SERVINGS

Chayote is a squash that is low in carbohydrates and rich in nutrients and antioxidants. It can be eaten raw. We love using chayote in our apple pie recipe. It takes on all the flavors you add to it and actually tastes like real apple pie after it's baked. You can also take the recipe for the filling a step further to make Chayote Applesauce (page 245).

IN a large bowl using a hand mixer, beat together the butter and cream cheese until smooth. Add one of the eggs and the salt and beat well. Add the almond flour, psyllium husk, tapioca starch, and xanthan gum and beat until combined.

DIVIDE the dough into two pieces, wrap in plastic wrap, and chill for at least 4 hours or overnight.

PREHEAT the oven to 350°F.

ON a sheet of parchment paper, roll out one piece of dough to a 13-inch round, about ¼ inch thick. Fit into an 8-inch pie plate, letting the extra dough overlap the edges. Using a fork, poke holes in the bottom of the pie crust. Spoon the chayote compote into the pie pan. Set aside.

ROLL out the remaining piece of dough into an 11-inch round and cut it into 1-inch-wide strips. Weave a lattice top with the strips of dough over the chayote compote. Trim the edges of the dough with a sharp knife and press the dough together with your thumbs and forefingers to seal the edges and create a decorative border.

IN a small bowl, mix together the remaining egg and 2 teaspoons water to make an egg wash. Brush the egg wash over the lattice crust.

BAKE for 15 to 18 minutes, until the crust is a golden brown on the edges.

NUTRITIONAL INFO (PER SERVING)
CALORIES 147, **FAT** 9g, **PROTEIN** 2.8g, **CARBS** 8.5g, **FIBER** 1.1g

STRAWBERRY PIE

STRAWBERRY FILLING

4 cups fresh strawberries, cut into quarters

²/₃ cup monkfruit powdered sweetener

2 packets True Lemon or 1 tablespoon lemon juice

½ teaspoon ground cinnamon

½ teaspoon xanthan gum

CRUST

2 cups shredded part-skim low-moisture mozzarella cheese

5 tablespoons butter, melted

2 large eggs

½ cup blanched almond flour

¼ cup coconut flour

1 tablespoon monkfruit powdered sweetener

1½ teaspoons baking powder

MAKES 2 (7-INCH) FREEFORM PIES (12 SERVINGS)

I love to make this when strawberries are in season, so our summers are full of rustic pie. It's pretty great topped with your favorite keto ice cream.

PREHEAT the oven to 350°F. Have a baking sheet ready.

FOR THE STRAWBERRY FILLING

IN a medium bowl, mix together the strawberries, sweetener, True Lemon, cinnamon, and xanthan gum. If your strawberries are not juicy, you may need to add 1 tablespoon water to the mixture, until it's loose but thick. Set aside.

FOR THE CRUST

IN a microwave-safe bowl, heat the mozzarella in the microwave oven for 1 to 1½ minutes until melted. Working quickly, immediately add the butter to the cheese and mix to combine. Add one of the eggs and mix to combine. Add the almond flour, coconut flour, sweetener, and baking powder and mix until it forms a stiff dough. Knead the dough until all the ingredients are combined. It will be sticky at first but the longer you knead, the stickiness will go away. If the dough has cooled too much and becomes stiff, heat it in the microwave oven for 30 seconds and continue to knead until combined. Divide the dough into two pieces.

ON sheets of parchment paper, roll out each piece of dough to a 12-inch round. Spoon half of the strawberry filling into the center of each dough circle. Fold over the edges of the dough just enough to create a border to hold the strawberry filling in. Transfer each pie to the baking sheet.

IN a small bowl, whisk together the remaining egg and 2 teaspoons water to make an egg wash. Brush the crust of both pies with the wash.

BAKE for 30 minutes, or until the crusts are golden brown.

NUTRITIONAL INFO (PER SERVING)
CALORIES 129, **FAT** 6.4g, **PROTEIN** 8g, **CARBS** 8g, **FIBER** 2.5g

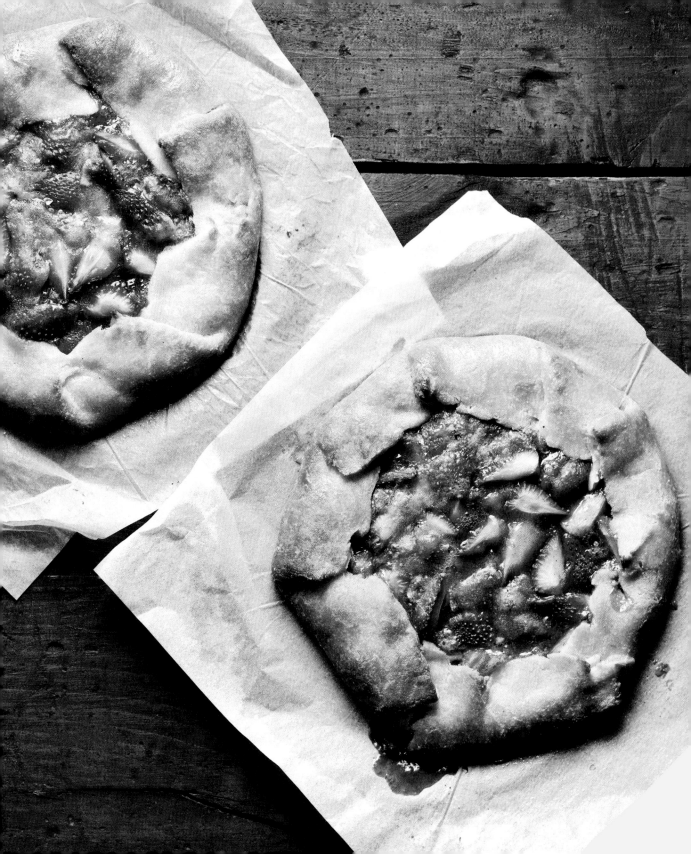

SUGAR-FREE GANACHE

½ cup heavy whipping cream

½ cup Lily's stevia-sweetened dark chocolate chips

MAKES 1 CUP (8 SERVINGS)

This is a quick and yummy sugar-free ganache that can be used to frost cookies or cakes. It's super easy to make when you use Lily's sugar-free chocolate chips because they are sweetened with stevia so the recipe requires only two ingredients.

IN a microwave-safe bowl, heat the cream in the microwave oven for 30 seconds, or until the cream is between 90°F and 110°F. Add the chocolate chips, cover the bowl, and let sit for 2 minutes. Carefully whisk the chocolate and cream together for about 1 minute, until smooth.

STORE in a covered container in the refrigerator for up to 2 weeks.

NUTRITIONAL INFO (PER 2-TABLESPOON SERVING)
CALORIES 51, **FAT** 5.4g, **PROTEIN** 0.4g, **CARBS** 0.4g, **FIBER** 0g

GANACHE RATIOS

1 part heavy cream + 2 parts chocolate = very thick ganache for truffles.

1 part heavy cream + 1 part chocolate = spreadable ganache for frosting or filling sweet treats.

2 parts heavy cream + 1 part chocolate = pourable ganache for cakes or glaze for doughnuts.

BUTTERCREAM FROSTING

16 tablespoons (2 sticks) butter

¾ cup monkfruit powdered sweetener

2 teaspoons heavy whipping cream

2 teaspoons almond extract

1 teaspoon vanilla extract

MAKES 2 CUPS (13 SERVINGS)

This buttercream has a hint of almond extract which adds an extra special flavor. Use it to frost cakes or cookies.

IN a large bowl using a hand mixer, beat the butter and sweetener until smooth. Add the cream, almond extract, and vanilla and beat until light and fluffy.

NUTRITIONAL INFO (PER 2½-TABLESPOON SERVING)
CALORIES 140, **FAT** 15.5g, **PROTEIN** 0.2g, **CARBS** 0.4g, **FIBER** 0g

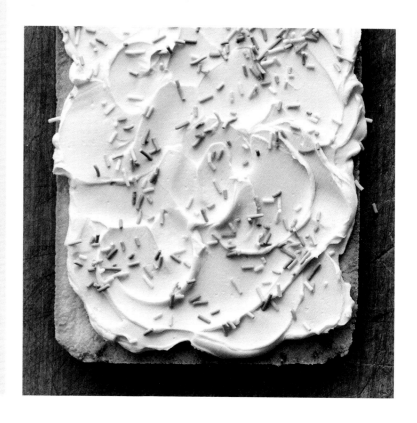

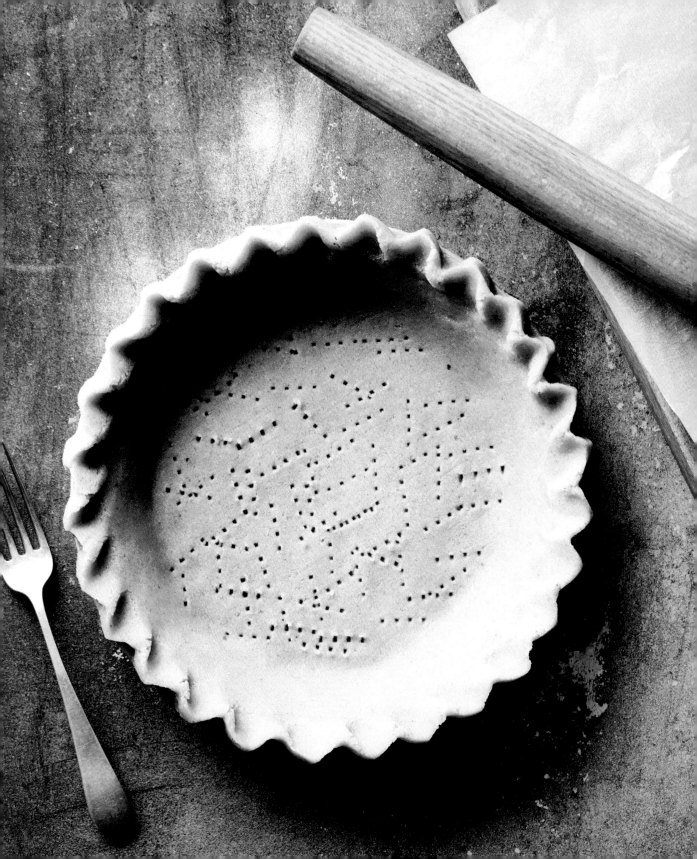

FLAKY PIE SHELL

12 tablespoons (1½ sticks)
  butter

2 ounces cream cheese

1 large egg

1 teaspoon salt

2 cups blanched almond flour

¼ cup coconut flour

2 tablespoons psyllium husk

2 tablespoons tapioca starch

¼ teaspoon xanthan gum

MAKES 2 (8-INCH) PIE SHELLS (16 SERVINGS)

What makes this pie crust so flaky is the high concentration of good fat—in this case, butter. In addition to the Pumpkin Pie (page 234), you can use the crust for other sweet pies and tarts and savory quiches. If you'd like to prebake the shell, bake in a 350°F oven for 13 to 15 minutes, until golden brown. Let cool for 15 minutes before filling.

IN a large bowl using a hand mixer, beat together the butter and cream cheese until smooth. Add the egg and salt and beat until combined. Add the almond flour, coconut flour, psyllium husk, tapioca starch, and xanthan gum and beat until combined.

DIVIDE the dough into two pieces, wrap in plastic wrap, and chill for at least 4 hours or overnight.

HAVE two 8-inch pie plates and one sheet of parchment paper ready.

ON the sheet of parchment paper, roll out one piece of dough to a 13-inch round, about ¼ inch thick. Fit it into an 8-inch pie plate, letting the extra dough overlap the edges. Using a fork, poke holes in the bottom of the pie crust. Trim the edges of the dough with a sharp knife and press the dough together with your thumbs and forefingers to create a decorative border. Repeat with the second piece of dough.

THE pie shells can be stored, wrapped tightly in plastic, in the refrigerator for 7 days or frozen for up to 3 months.

NUTRITIONAL INFO (PER SERVING)
CALORIES 181, **FAT** 12.8g, **PROTEIN** 3.1g, **CARBS** 4g, **FIBER** 1.2g

SAVORY PIE SHELL

12 tablespoons (1½ sticks) butter

2 ounces cream cheese

1 large egg

1 teaspoon salt

2 cups blanched almond flour

¼ cup coconut flour

2 tablespoons psyllium husk

2 tablespoons tapioca starch

1 teaspoon dried parsley

1 teaspoon onion powder

½ teaspoon dried dill

¼ teaspoon xanthan gum

MAKES 2 (8-INCH) PIE SHELLS (16 SERVINGS TOTAL)

I've included this savory crust because it's perfect to use when making the Cheeseburger Pie (page 116) and the Sausage Quiche (page 125). To prebake the shell, bake at 350°F for 13 to 15 minutes, until golden brown. Let cool for 15 minutes before filling.

IN a large bowl using a hand mixer, beat together the butter and cream cheese until smooth. Add the egg and salt and beat until combined. Add the almond flour, coconut flour, psyllium husk, tapioca starch, parsley, onion powder, dill, and xanthan gum and beat to combine.

DIVIDE the dough into two pieces, wrap in plastic wrap, and chill for at least 4 hours or overnight.

HAVE two 8-inch pie plates and a sheet of parchment paper ready.

ON the sheet of parchment paper, roll out one piece of dough to a 13-inch round, about ¼ inch thick. Fit it into one pie plate, letting the extra dough overlap the edges. Using a fork, poke holes in the bottom of the pie crust. Trim the edges of the dough with a sharp knife and press the dough together with your thumbs and forefingers to create a decorative border. Repeat with the second piece of dough.

THE pie shells can be stored, wrapped tightly in plastic, in the refrigerator for 7 days or frozen for up to 3 months.

NUTRITIONAL INFO (PER SERVING)
CALORIES 185, **FAT** 12.8g, **PROTEIN** 3.1g, **CARBS** 4.9g, **FIBER** 1.2g

CHAYOTE APPLESAUCE

3 chayote squash, peeled, seeded, and chopped

1 teaspoon ground cinnamon

¼ cup monkfruit sweetener

1 teaspoon lemon juice

2 tablespoons Swerve brown sugar sweetener

1 teaspoon butter

¼ teaspoon maple extract

MAKES 2 PINTS (8 SERVINGS)

When you are living a keto way of life and can't eat a lot of fruit, like apples, I love it when I find an alternate that satisfies my craving. I no longer miss applesauce because this version made with chayote squash tastes very similar to the original.

INSTANT POT METHOD: Place a steamer basket in an Instant Pot and pour in 1 cup water. Place the chopped chayote and cinnamon in the pot and seal with the lid. Press the manual setting and set it to high pressure for 20 minutes. When the cycle ends, perform a quick release.

DRAIN the chayote in a strainer and set aside.

IN a large skillet over medium heat, mix together the chayote, monkfruit sweetener, and lemon juice and cook, stirring frequently until the liquid has reduced. Add the brown sugar sweetener, butter, and maple extract and continue to cook for 5 more minutes, until the mixture appears caramelized like caramel sauce. Let cool.

STOVETOP METHOD: In a large skillet over medium-high heat, mix together the chayote, cinnamon, and 4 cups water and bring to a boil. Reduce the heat to medium-low and simmer, adding more water as needed, until the chayote is soft, 35 to 40 minutes.

ADD the monkfruit sweetener and lemon juice and continue to cook, stirring frequently, until most of the liquid has reduced. Add the brown sugar sweetener, butter, and maple extract and continue to cook for about 5 more minutes, until the mixture appears caramelized like caramel sauce. Let cool.

TO FINISH: Transfer the chayote mixture to a blender and blend until it has the texture of applesauce. Serve immediately or store in a covered container and refrigerate for up to 5 days.

NUTRITIONAL INFO (PER SERVING)
CALORIES 15, **FAT** 1.5g, **PROTEIN** 0.2g, **CARBS** 0.9g, **FIBER** 0.2g

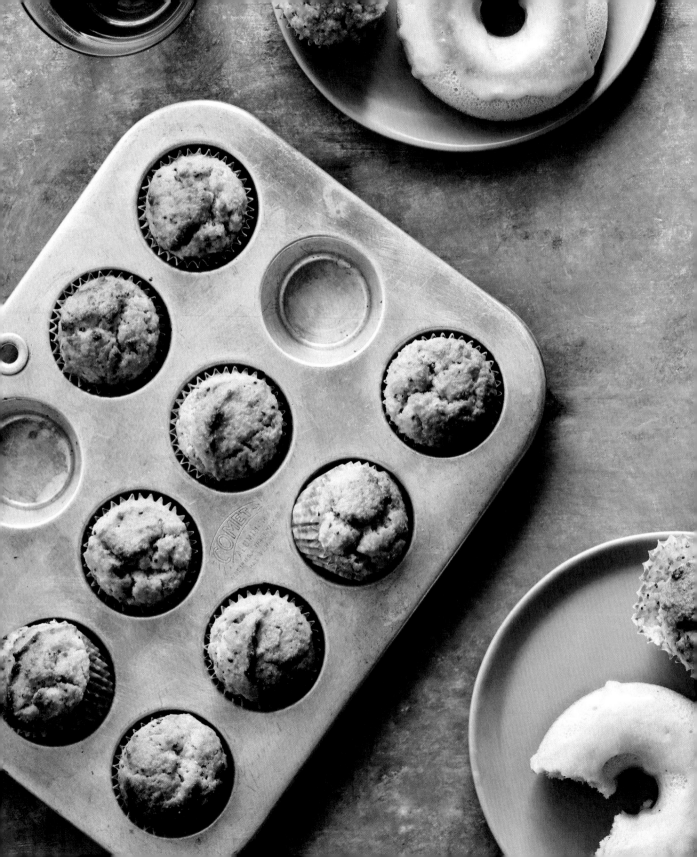

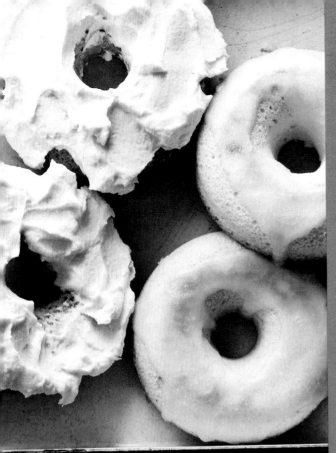

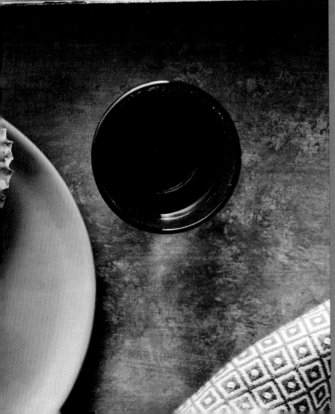

MUFFINS, DOUGHNUTS, & OTHER SWEET TREATS

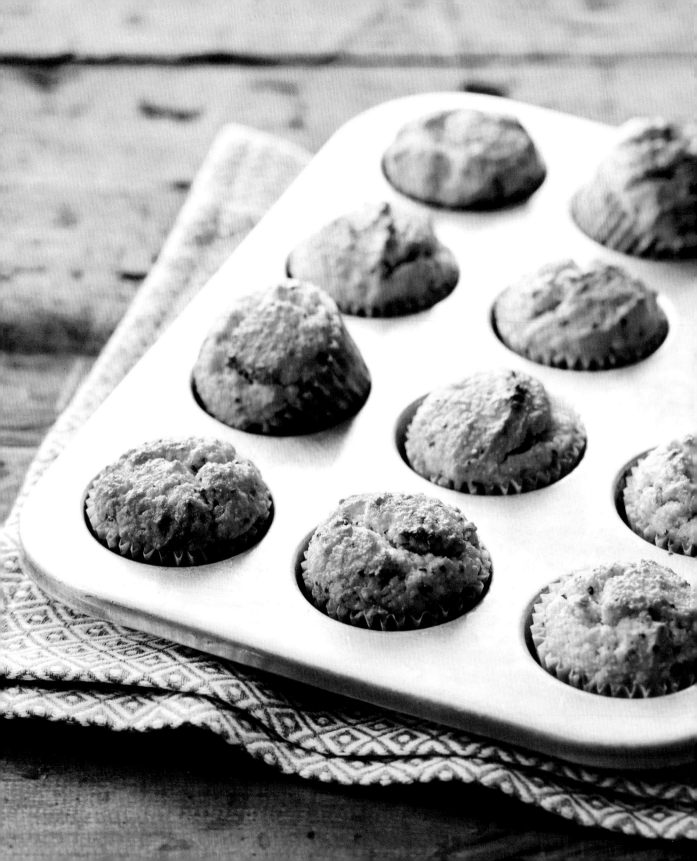

LEMON–CHIA SEED MUFFINS

4 ounces cream cheese, at room temperature

4 large eggs, at room temperature

1 teaspoon grated lemon zest

2 tablespoons lemon juice

1 teaspoon vanilla extract

1¼ cups blanched almond flour

¾ cup Swerve confectioners' sweetener

4 tablespoons butter, at room temperature

2 tablespoons coconut flour

2 tablespoons whole chia seeds

1 tablespoon ground chia seeds

1½ teaspoons unflavored collagen peptides

¾ teaspoon baking powder

½ teaspoon salt

MAKES 12 MUFFINS

Packed with fiber and the sweet-tart taste of lemon, I often make a double batch of these muffins to take on road trips.

PREHEAT the oven to 350°F. Line the cups of a 12-cup muffin tin with cupcake liners and spray the liners with nonstick cooking spray.

IN a medium bowl using a hand mixer, beat the cream cheese, eggs, lemon zest, lemon juice, and vanilla until combined. Add the almond flour, sweetener, butter, coconut flour, whole chia, ground chia, collagen peptides, baking powder, and salt and beat until combined.

USE an ice cream scoop to spoon the mixture equally into the muffin cups. Bake for 30 to 35 minutes, until a toothpick inserted into the center of a muffin comes out clean.

NUTRITIONAL INFO (PER MUFFIN)
CALORIES 92, **FAT** 6g, **PROTEIN** 2.8g, **CARBS** 7.3g, **FIBER** 1g

TRIPLE-BERRY MUFFINS

4 ounces cream cheese, at room temperature

4 large eggs, at room temperature

1 teaspoon grated lemon zest

2 tablespoons lemon juice

1 teaspoon lemon extract

1 teaspoon vanilla extract

1¼ cups blanched almond flour

¾ cups Swerve confectioners' sweetener

4 tablespoons butter

2 tablespoons coconut flour

¾ teaspoon baking powder

½ teaspoon salt

1½ cups chopped fresh berries (strawberries, blueberries, raspberries)

MAKES 12 MUFFINS

There are not many fruits of the keto diet, but berries make the cut, so I created this triple threat of a muffin and make them all the time. Have them for breakfast, a snack, or pack them up and take them on the go.

PREHEAT the oven to 350°F. Line the cups of a 12-cup muffin tin with cupcake liners and spray the liners with nonstick cooking spray.

IN a medium bowl using a hand mixer, beat the cream cheese, eggs, lemon zest, lemon juice, lemon extract, and vanilla until combined. Add the almond flour, sweetener, butter, coconut flour, baking powder, and salt and beat until combined. Fold in the berries.

USE an ice cream scoop to spoon the mixture equally into the muffin cups. Bake for 30 to 35 minutes, until a toothpick inserted into the center of a muffin comes out clean.

NUTRITIONAL INFO (PER MUFFIN)
CALORIES 176, **FAT** 11g, **PROTEIN** 4.8g, **CARBS** 6.8g, **FIBER** 1.3g

PUMPKIN CHAFFLES

PUMPKIN CHAFFLES

1 large egg

½ cup shredded part-skim low-moisture mozzarella cheese

1 tablespoon pure pumpkin puree

½ teaspoon pumpkin pie spice

CREAM CHEESE FROSTING

2 tablespoons cream cheese, at room temperature

2 tablespoons monkfruit powdered sweetener

½ teaspoon clear vanilla extract

MAKES 2 CHAFFLES

This recipe uses a small amount of pumpkin, so I always have some leftover. But that's okay, because I can freeze it in small covered containers for up to 4 months to have whenever I need it.

FOR THE PUMPKIN CHAFFLES

PREHEAT a mini waffle maker according to the manufacturer's instructions.

IN a small bowl, whisk the egg. Add the mozzarella cheese, pumpkin puree, and pumpkin pie spice and mix to combine.

SPOON half of the batter into the waffle maker and cook for 3 to 4 minutes, until golden brown. Repeat with the remaining batter. Transfer the chaffles to serving plates.

FOR THE CREAM CHEESE FROSTING

IN a small bowl using a hand mixer, beat the cream cheese, sweetener, and vanilla until smooth. Spread the frosting over the hot chaffles and serve immediately.

NUTRITIONAL INFO (PER CHAFFLE)
CALORIES 67, **FAT** 3.7g, **PROTEIN** 6.5g, **CARBS** 3.5g, **FIBER** 0.4g

FROSTED PUMPKIN DOUGHNUTS

DOUGHNUTS

2 cups blanched almond flour

¾ cup monkfruit powdered sweetener

2 tablespoons unflavored collagen peptides

2 teaspoons ground cinnamon

1 teaspoon baking powder

¼ teaspoon ground ginger

¼ teaspoon ground nutmeg

¼ teaspoon salt

4 large eggs

¼ cup pure pumpkin puree

2 teaspoons vanilla extract

CREAM CHEESE FROSTING

8 ounces cream cheese, at room temperature

8 tablespoons (1 stick) butter, at room temperature

½ cup monkfruit powdered sweetener

2 teaspoons vanilla extract

MAKES 12 MINI DOUGHNUTS

You'll fool your friends with these doughnuts. The texture is so like a classic doughnut that even if you tell them the doughnuts are keto friendly, they might not believe you. The collagen peptides are a wonderful way to add extra protein and it's the secret ingredient that makes each doughnut super moist and delicious. Don't even think of leaving it out!

FOR THE DOUGHNUTS

PREHEAT the oven to 350°F. Grease 12 cups of a silicone mini doughnut mold and place on a baking sheet.

IN a large bowl, combine the almond flour, sweetener, collagen peptides, cinnamon, baking powder, ginger, nutmeg, and salt.

IN a medium bowl, whisk the eggs until frothy. Add the pumpkin and vanilla and mix to combine. Add the pumpkin mixture to the almond flour mixture and mix until fully combined.

USING a piping bag or a zip-top bag, pipe the batter into the doughnut molds. Bake for 22 to 25 minutes, until golden brown and a toothpick inserted into a doughnut comes out clean. Transfer the doughnuts to a wire rack to cool completely.

FOR THE CREAM CHEESE FROSTING

IN a medium bowl using a hand mixer, beat the cream cheese, butter, sweetener, and vanilla until smooth.

SPREAD the frosting on the cooled doughnuts and serve.

NUTRITIONAL INFO (PER MINI DOUGHNUT)
CALORIES 280, **FAT** 19.1g, **PROTEIN** 7.9g, **CARBS** 6.3g, **FIBER** 1.1g

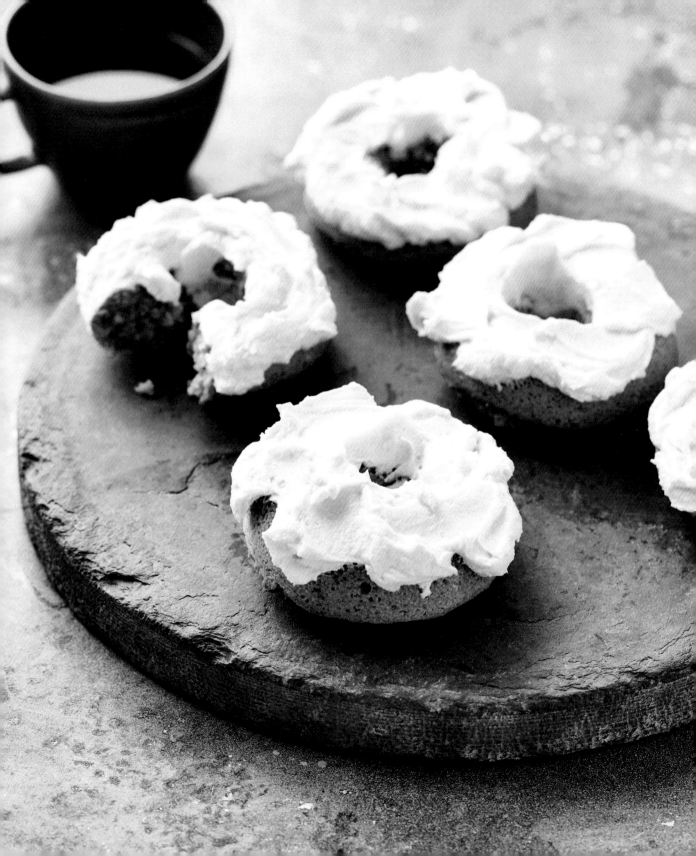

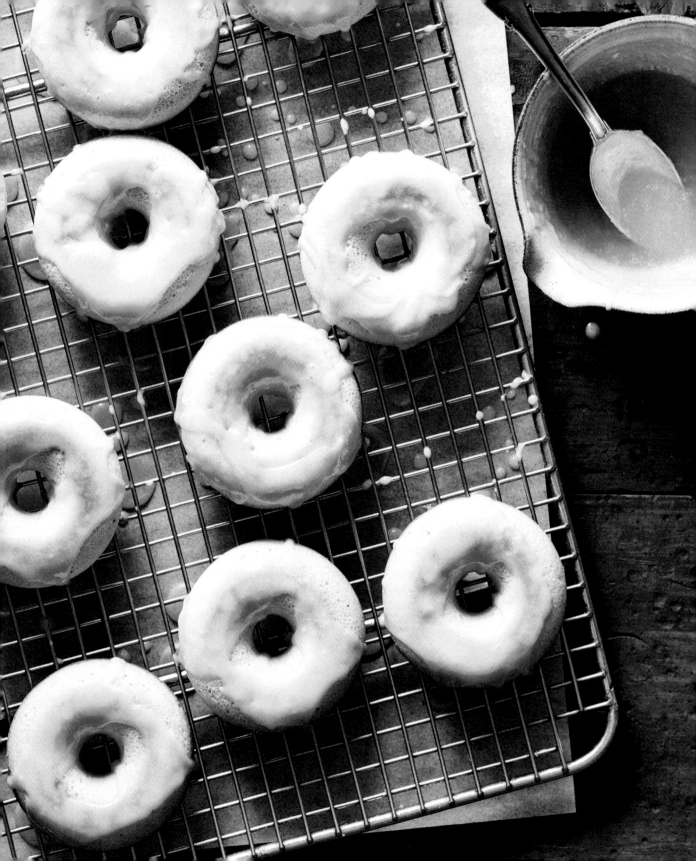

SOUR CREAM DOUGHNUTS

DOUGHNUTS

2 cups blanched almond flour

¾ cup monkfruit powdered sweetener

2 tablespoons unflavored collagen peptides

1 teaspoon baking powder

½ teaspoon ground nutmeg

2 large eggs

4 large egg whites or ½ cup liquid egg whites

½ cup sour cream

GLAZE

4 tablespoons butter

¼ cup monkfruit powdered sweetener

2 tablespoons heavy whipping cream

1 teaspoon vanilla extract

MAKES 12 MINI DOUGHNUTS

One of the things I love about the keto diet is that I can eat things like these indulgent doughnuts and don't need to feel deprived. The collagen peptides are what make these doughnuts super-moist and delicious.

FOR THE DOUGHNUTS

PREHEAT the oven to 350°F. Grease 12 cups of a silicone mini doughnut mold and place on a baking sheet.

IN a medium bowl, mix together the almond flour, sweetener, collagen peptides, baking powder, and nutmeg.

IN a separate medium bowl, whisk the eggs and egg whites until frothy. Add the sour cream and mix to combine. Add the egg mixture to the almond flour mixture and mix until fully combined.

USING a piping bag or zip-top bag, pipe the batter into the doughnut molds. Bake for 22 to 25 minutes, until golden brown and a toothpick inserted into a doughnut comes out clean. Transfer the doughnuts to a wire rack to cool completely.

FOR THE GLAZE

IN a small saucepan over medium heat, melt the butter. Add the sweetener and cream and bring to a simmer, stirring frequently, until slightly thickened, about 5 minutes. Stir in the vanilla.

DRIZZLE the hot glaze over the doughnuts and serve.

NUTRITIONAL INFO (PER MINI DOUGHNUT)
CALORIES 264, **FAT** 18.1g, **PROTEIN** 7.1g, **CARBS** 5.5g, **FIBER** 0.7g

PEANUT BUTTER WAFFLES

PEANUT BUTTER WAFFLES

1 large egg

2 tablespoons sugar-free peanut butter powder

2 tablespoons monkfruit powdered sweetener

1 tablespoon heavy whipping cream

¼ teaspoon baking powder

¼ teaspoon LorAnn peanut butter flavoring

PEANUT BUTTER FROSTING

2 tablespoons cream cheese, at room temperature

2 tablespoons monkfruit powdered sweetener

1 tablespoon butter, at room temperature

1 tablespoon sugar-free natural peanut butter or peanut butter powder

¼ teaspoon vanilla extract

MAKES 4 WAFFLES

For an intense peanut butter flavor, make sure to use the peanut butter flavoring. But if you can't find it easily, it's fine to make the waffles without it. The flavor will just be a more subtle.

FOR THE PEANUT BUTTER WAFFLES

PREHEAT a mini waffle maker according to the manufacturer's instructions.

IN a small bowl, whisk the egg. Add the peanut butter powder, sweetener, cream, baking powder, and peanut butter flavoring and mix until smooth.

POUR half of the batter into the waffle maker and cook for 2 to 3 minutes, until browned. Repeat with the remaining batter. Let the waffles cool completely.

FOR THE PEANUT BUTTER FROSTING

IN a small bowl, mix together the cream cheese, sweetener, butter, peanut butter, and vanilla until smooth. Spread the frosting on the waffles and serve.

VARIATIONS

PIPE IT: Use a piping bag or zip-top bag to pipe the frosting decoratively onto the waffles.

DRIZZLE IT: Add ½ teaspoon water to the frosting ingredients and mix until smooth. Drizzle the peanut butter glaze over the waffles and serve.

NUTRITIONAL INFO (PER WAFFLE)
CALORIES 130, **FAT** 12.1g, **PROTEIN** 3.9g, **CARBS** 5g, **FIBER** 0.5g

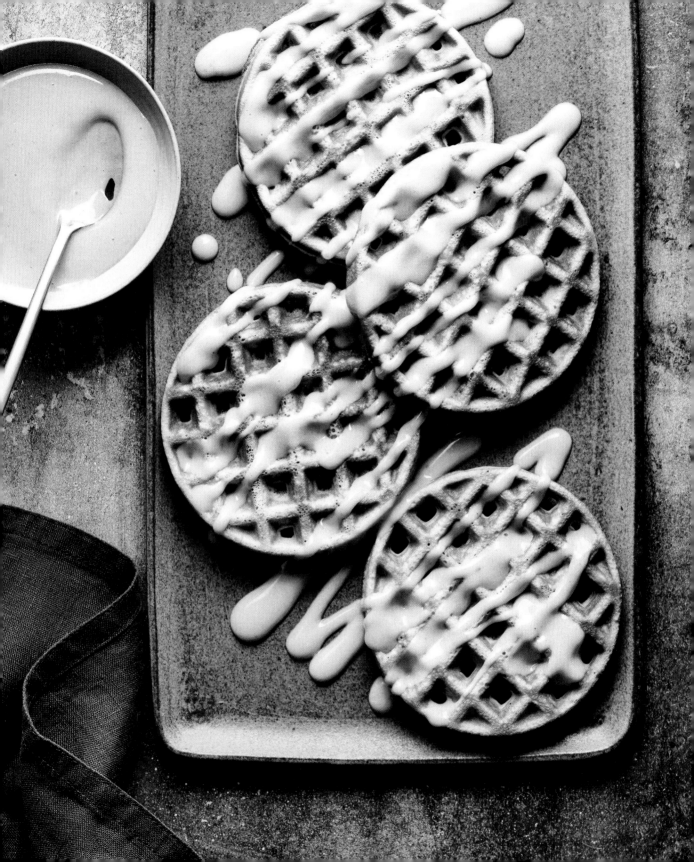

CREAM HORNS

PASTRY

1¾ cups shredded part-skim low-moisture mozzarella cheese

¾ cup blanched almond flour

2 tablespoons cream cheese, at room temperature

1 large egg

2 tablespoons Swerve confectioners' sweetener

½ teaspoon vanilla extract

WHIPPED CREAM FILLING

1 cup heavy whipping cream

1 tablespoon Swerve confectioners' sweetener

1 teaspoon vanilla extract

Blueberries, strawberries, or raspberries, optional

MAKES 12 CREAM HORNS

For a dessert that is special enough for the holidays, keto friendly, and completely delicious, you can't go wrong with cream horns. I like to make a double batch because everyone loves them. You will need cream horn molds to make these in the perfect shape, but they are inexpensive and easy to find online.

FOR THE PASTRY

PREHEAT the oven to 350°F. Have two sheets of parchment paper ready. Spray 12 (5-inch) cream horn molds with cooking spray and wrap pieces of parchment paper around them. Line a baking sheet with parchment paper or a silicone mat and place the prepared molds on the baking sheet.

IN a microwave-safe bowl, mix together the mozzarella, almond flour, and cream cheese and heat in the microwave oven for 1 minute. Add the egg, sweetener, and vanilla and mix until combined. The dough will be sticky. Let the dough cool for 1 to 2 minutes before handling.

DIVIDE the dough into two equal pieces. Place one piece on one sheet of parchment. Place the second piece of parchment on top. Using a rolling pin, roll out the dough to about 15 inches, ¼ inch thick. The dough will seem sticky at first but it will come together as you roll. Using a pizza cutter, cut 5-inch-wide strips of dough large enough to cover the cream horn molds. Wrap the strips of dough around the molds and place them on the baking sheet.

BAKE for 12 to 15 minutes, until golden brown. Transfer the baking sheet to a wire rack and let cool completely before removing the pastry from the molds.

FOR THE WHIPPED CREAM FILLING

IN a medium bowl using a hand mixer, beat the cream, sweetener, and vanilla on high, until stiff peaks form, about 5 minutes. Transfer the filling to a piping bag or a large zip-top bag. Fill each cream horn with filling and top each with berries, if using.

NUTRITIONAL INFO (PER SERVING)
CALORIES 93, **FAT** 8.6g, **PROTEIN** 4.9g, **CARBS** 2.7g, **FIBER** 0.2g

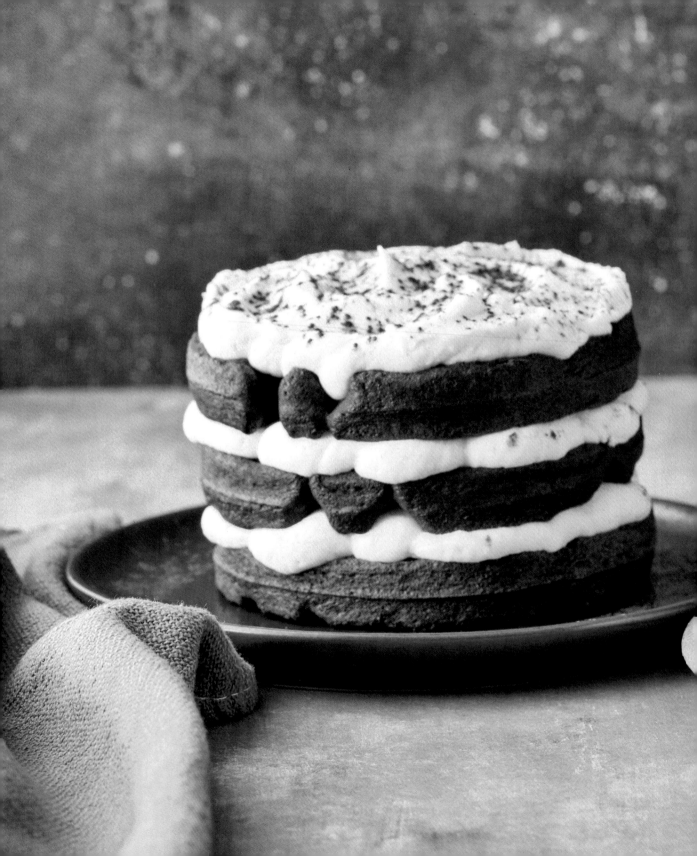

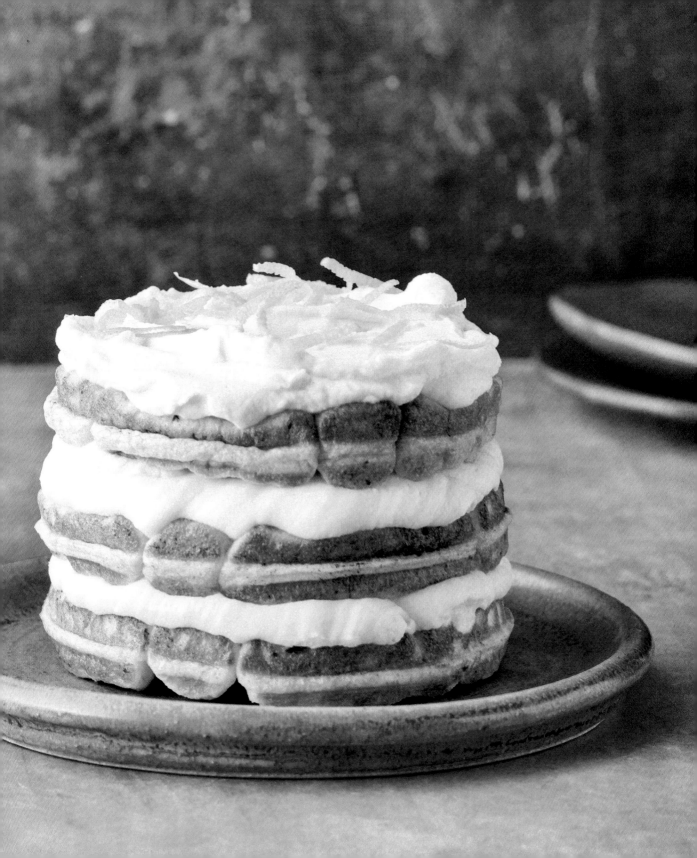

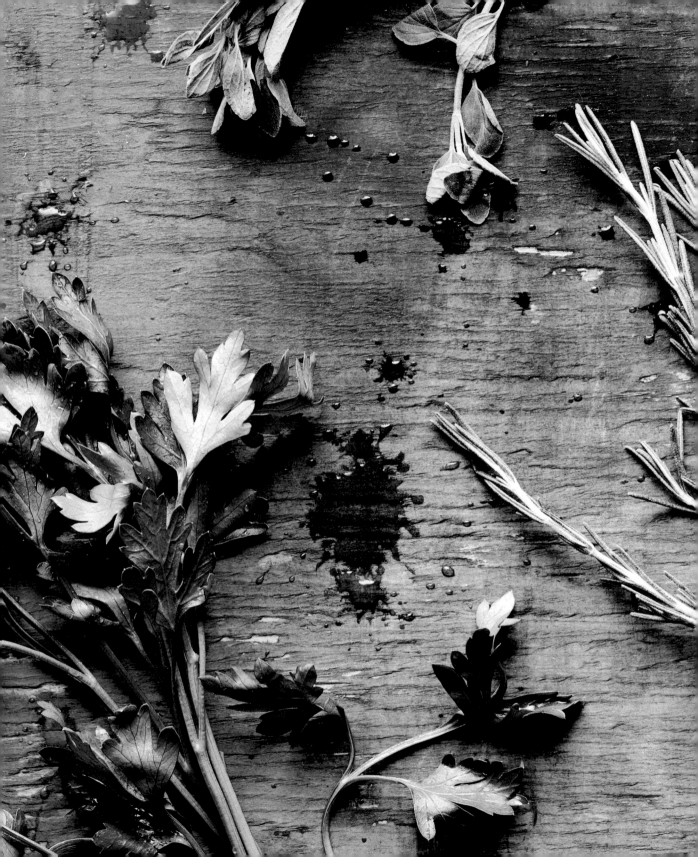

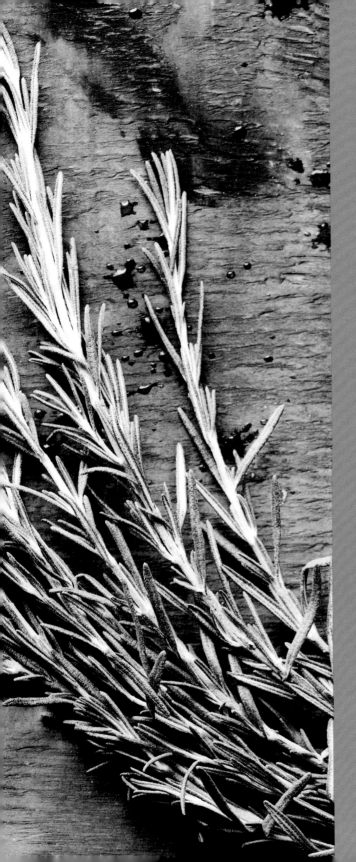

KETO BASICS

STOVETOP CHICKEN STOCK

2 to 4 pounds raw or roasted chicken bones

1 onion, peel on, trimmed and chopped into large chunks

2 stalks celery, coarsely chopped

2 tablespoons apple cider vinegar

1 tablespoon pink Himalayan salt

2 sprigs fresh rosemary

MAKES 5 QUARTS

Chicken stock is a fantastic base for so many recipes, and homemade always tastes the best. Even better, making stock is a great way to make use of leftover chicken bones. The next time you make dinner with bone-in chicken, save the bones in a zip-top bag in the freezer. When you accumulate 2 to 4 pounds, it's a good day to make stock.

COMBINE 5 quarts water and the chicken bones, onion, celery, vinegar, salt, and rosemary in a large soup pot. Bring to a boil over high heat. Lower the heat and simmer for at least 6 hours or up to 12 hours. Skim off any foam that forms during the first couple hours of cooking. Stir occasionally and add water as needed; the water should cover the bones completely.

STRAIN the stock into a large bowl and discard the solids. Let the stock cool.

STORE the cooled stock in a covered container in the refrigerator for up to 4 days, or in the freezer for up to 4 months. Be sure to leave a little extra room at the top of the container to allow for expansion as the stock freezes.

NUTRITIONAL INFO (PER 1 CUP)
CALORIES 8, **FAT** 0.1g, **PROTEIN** 1g, **CARBS** 0.9g, **FIBER** 0.2g

Notes: *Roasted bones create even richer, deeper flavor. Save any bones left over from your meals and roast in a 400°F oven for 15 minutes, until they become a dark brown, then use in the recipe. Be sure to also save any vegetable trimmings or scraps for stock. Simply toss them into the pot along with the other ingredients. It's a great way to use the parts you would normally throw away.*

PRESSURE COOKER BONE BROTH

2 to 4 pounds chicken or beef bones

1 onion, trimmed but left whole

2 stalks celery

2 tablespoons apple cider vinegar

2 sprigs fresh rosemary

1 tablespoon pink Himalayan salt

MAKES 15 CUPS

Bone broth is important when you are doing the keto diet because it provides tons of minerals and the electrolytes you need. I make it a point to drink a cup a day with a dab of butter and an extra sprinkle of salt on top. You may end up with more or less than 15 cups, depending on the size of your pressure cooker and how much liquid it can hold.

PREHEAT the oven to 400°F.

PLACE all the bones on a large baking sheet and roast for 30 minutes, until dark brown.

TRANSFER the bones to the pressure cooker. Add the onion, celery, vinegar, rosemary, salt, and enough water to reach the fill line of the cooker. Select the soup button, set the pressure to low, and increase the time setting to 120 minutes.

AFTER cooking, let the cooker naturally release the pressure. Strain the broth into a large bowl and discard the solids. Let the broth cool.

STORE in a covered container in the refrigerator for up to 4 days, or in the freezer for up to 4 months. Be sure to leave a little extra room at the top of the container to allow for expansion as the broth freezes.

NUTRITIONAL INFO (PER 1 CUP)
CALORIES 34, **FAT** 1g, **PROTEIN** 1.5g, **CARBS** 4.9g, **FIBER** 0.8g

BASIC CONDENSED CREAM SOUP

10 ounces cooked chicken or drained canned chicken

½ cup heavy whipping cream

2 ounces cream cheese, at room temperature

2 tablespoons butter, at room temperature

¼ teaspoon paprika

¼ teaspoon onion powder

¼ teaspoon garlic powder

MAKES 1½ CUPS (3 SERVINGS)

This is a super-thick homemade version of canned condensed soup that I use as a base for soups and as an addition to casseroles. Add 1 cup Pressure Cooker Bone Broth (page 265) to use it as a soup base.

IN a blender, mix the chicken, cream, cream cheese, butter, paprika, onion powder, and garlic powder and blend on high for 20 seconds, or until smooth. The mixture will be very thick.

TRANSFER the mixture to a medium saucepan and cook over medium heat, stirring, until heated through, 3 to 5 minutes.

VARIATIONS

BURRITO SAUCE: Add 1 (4-ounce) can of green chiles.

SPICY SAUCE: Add 1 (10-ounce) can of Ro*Tel diced tomatoes and green chilies and pour the sauce over chicken.

MUSHROOM SOUP: Cook ½ pound sliced mushrooms in 2 tablespoons butter, stirring. Add to the cream soup along with 1 cup bone broth and heat to simmering.

NUTRITIONAL INFO (PER ½ CUP)
CALORIES 357, **FAT** 26g, **PROTEIN** 27.9g, **CARBS** 2g, **FIBER** 0.1g

BASIC DAIRY-FREE CONDENSED SOUP

10 ounces cooked chicken or drained canned chicken

1 (13½-ounce) can unsweetened coconut milk

½ teaspoon paprika

½ teaspoon onion powder

½ teaspoon garlic powder

½ teaspoon salt

MAKES 2½ CUPS

This is a dairy-free version of condensed cream soup that can be used for those who are lactose-intolerant. The soup does have a slight coconut taste, so make sure you use it with flavors that pair well with coconut. Use it as a layer in a casserole, or add 1 cup bone broth to make it a soup base.

IN a blender, mix together the chicken, coconut milk, paprika, onion powder, garlic powder, and salt. Blend on high for 20 seconds, or until combined. This mixture will be somewhat clumpy because of the fat content of the coconut milk.

TRANSFER the mixture to a medium saucepan and cook over medium heat, stirring, until heated through, 3 to 5 minutes.

NUTRITIONAL INFO (PER ½ CUP)
CALORIES 306, **FAT** 21g, **PROTEIN** 27.7g, **CARBS** 3g, **FIBER** 0.2g

Note: *You can use the same variations from the Basic Condensed Cream Soup (page 266).*

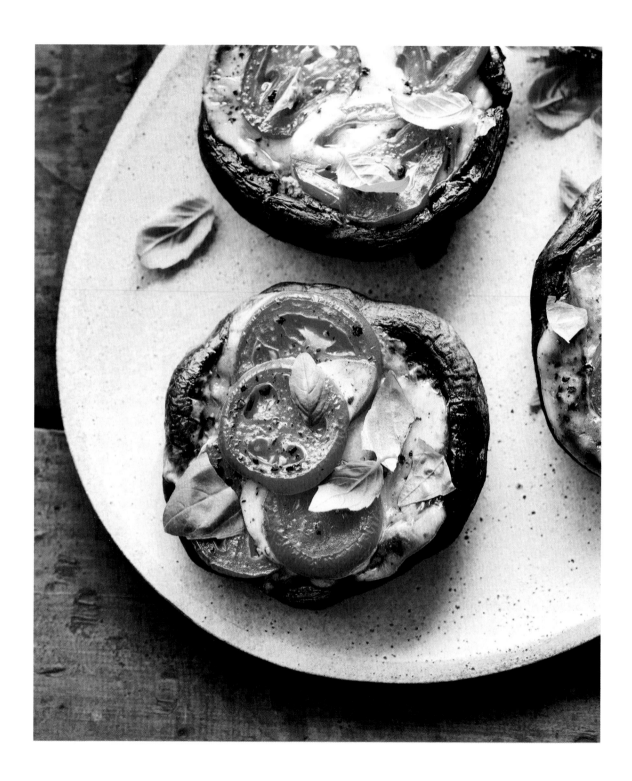

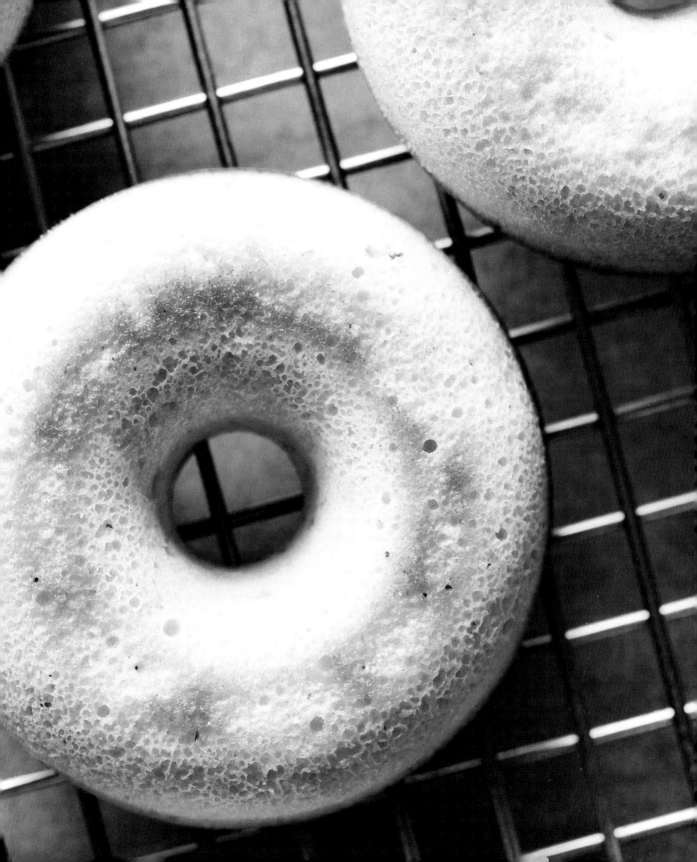

MAKIN' BACON

1 pound bacon

Save time in the kitchen and cook bacon ahead of time just before your week starts. I always save the bacon fat and use it in almost any recipe that requires oil, especially vegetables. When microwaving bacon (see Note), cook only a few pieces at a time.

PREHEAT the oven to 350°F. Line a baking sheet with aluminum foil and place a baking rack on top.

LAY the strips of bacon on the rack. Cover the bacon with a piece of parchment paper to prevent the oil from splattering.

BAKE for 30 to 40 minutes, depending on the thickness of the bacon and the desired crispiness. Reserve the fat for future use.

PLACE leftover bacon in a zip-top bag and refrigerate for up to 7 days or freeze for up to 6 months. To store bacon fat, pour it into an ice cube tray and freeze. When frozen, pop them out of the tray, transfer to a zip-top bag, and keep in the freezer until ready to use. One bacon fat ice cube is a nice portion to use in most recipes.

NUTRITIONAL INFO (PER SLICE)
CALORIES 117, **FAT** 11.1g, **PROTEIN** 3.5g, **CARBS** 0.4g, **FIBER** 0g

Note: If you don't want to bake a big batch of bacon, you can microwave 3 or 4 strips: Lay the strips on a microwave-safe plate and microwave on high for 3 minutes. Let cool slightly before using.

PULLED PORK

4 pounds pork shoulder

2 tablespoons All Seasoning Spice (page 274)

2 tablespoons extra-virgin olive oil

1 tablespoon apple cider vinegar

AlternaSweets original BBQ sauce, optional

MAKES 8 SERVINGS

Everyone needs a go-to pulled pork recipe and this one cooks up fast in an Instant Pot. Use it in the Cowboy Pork Casserole (page 123) or pile it on a chaffle.

IF the pork shoulder is too big for your pressure cooker, cut it into two pieces. Rub the pork with the All Seasoning.

PRESS the sauté setting on the pressure cooker. When hot, add the olive oil. Add the pork and brown for 3 to 4 minutes on each side. Transfer the pork to a plate.

TURN off the Instant Pot. Pour ½ cup water into the Instant Pot and deglaze by using a wooden spoon to scrape the brown bits off the bottom of the pot. Add the vinegar and return the pork to the Instant Pot.

PRESS the manual setting and set it to high pressure for 55 minutes. If your pork shoulder is larger than 4 pounds, add 5 minutes for every additional pound. When the cycle ends, let the pressure release naturally for 10 minutes. Transfer the pork to a cutting board and shred the meat using two forks. Serve immediately with the barbecue sauce, if using.

STORE in a covered container in the refrigerator for up to 4 days or freeze for up to 3 months.

NUTRITIONAL INFO (PER SERVING)
CALORIES 107, **FAT** 5.7g, **PROTEIN** 12.9g, **CARBS** 1g, **FIBER** 0.7g

BASIC FATHEAD DOUGH

1¾ cups shredded part-skim low-moisture mozzarella cheese

¾ cup blanched almond flour

2 tablespoons cream cheese

1 large egg

1 teaspoon dried rosemary, optional

MAKES ENOUGH DOUGH FOR 2 (12-INCH) PIZZA CRUSTS (16 SERVINGS)

I use this recipe all the time and I'll make several batches at a time and freeze to use later. The recipe gives instructions for using it to make pizza crust (as for the Club Pizza with Cold Ranch Salad on page 131), but you can also use it to make crackers, tortillas, bagels, calzones, dumplings, and rolls. The recipe here gives instructions for using it to make pizza crust.

PREHEAT the oven to 350°F. Have four large sheets of parchment paper and two baking sheets ready.

IN a microwave-safe bowl, combine the mozzarella, almond flour, and cream cheese and heat in the microwave oven until the cheese melts, about 1 minute. Mix together until completely combined. Add the egg and the rosemary, if using, and mix until a sticky, stiff dough forms. Let cool for about 5 minutes. Divide the dough into two pieces.

PLACE one piece of dough on one sheet of parchment and lay a second piece of parchment over the top. Using a rolling pin, roll out the dough to a 12-inch round. Slide the parchment paper with the dough onto the baking sheet. Repeat with the second piece of dough.

TO MAKE PIZZAS: Arrange whatever toppings you prefer on the dough and bake for 12 to 15 minutes, until the crust is golden brown and the toppings are hot. Slide the parchment paper onto a cooling rack and let the pizza cool for 5 minutes before cutting into slices.

TO store the unrolled dough, wrap in plastic wrap and refrigerate for up to 1 week, or freeze for up to 6 weeks. To defrost, place the ball of dough in the refrigerator for at least 24 hours. You may need to heat the dough in the microwave oven for 10 to 20 seconds to make it pliable enough to shape it the way you want.

TO freeze the rolled out dough, stack layers of the uncooked dough between sheets of parchment paper, place on a baking sheet, and wrap in plastic wrap. Freeze for up to 6 weeks. To defrost, let the dough sit at room temperature for about 20 minutes.

NUTRITIONAL INFO (PER SERVING)
CALORIES 126, **FAT** 9.8, **PROTEIN** 6.8g, **CARBS** 3.9g, **FIBER** 1.1g

ALL SEASONING SPICE

¼ cup pink Himalayan salt

2 teaspoons black pepper

1 teaspoon garlic powder

1 teaspoon onion powder

1 teaspoon paprika

1 teaspoon chili powder

¼ teaspoon ground cayenne pepper

¼ teaspoon ground celery seed

¼ teaspoon nutmeg

MAKES ABOUT 6 TABLESPOONS (24 SERVINGS)

Here is a basic combination of spices that you can use whenever you want a little added flavor. I call for pink Himalayan salt because it contains 84 minerals that are great for our bodies.

COMBINE all the ingredients in a bowl and mix until fully combined. Store in a covered container at room temperature for up to 2 years.

NUTRITIONAL INFO (PER 1 TEASPOON)
CALORIES 2, **FAT** 0.1g, **PROTEIN** 0.1g, **CARBS** 0.4g, **FIBER** 0.2g

TACO SEASONING

1 tablespoon chili powder

1 teaspoon unsweetened cocoa powder

¾ teaspoon ground cumin

½ teaspoon salt

½ teaspoon dried oregano

¼ teaspoon garlic powder

¼ teaspoon onion powder

MAKES ABOUT 3 TABLESPOONS (12 SERVINGS)

It's always best to make your own taco seasoning because most of the store-bought brands contain sugar. The cocoa powder adds a depth of flavor without a prominent taste of chocolate. It's a secret ingredient!

IN a small bowl, mix together all the ingredients. Store in a covered container at room temperature for up to 12 months.

NUTRITIONAL INFO (PER ¾ TEASPOON)
CALORIES 26, **FAT** 1.2g, **PROTEIN** 1.3g, **CARBS** 4.9g, **FIBER** 2.7g

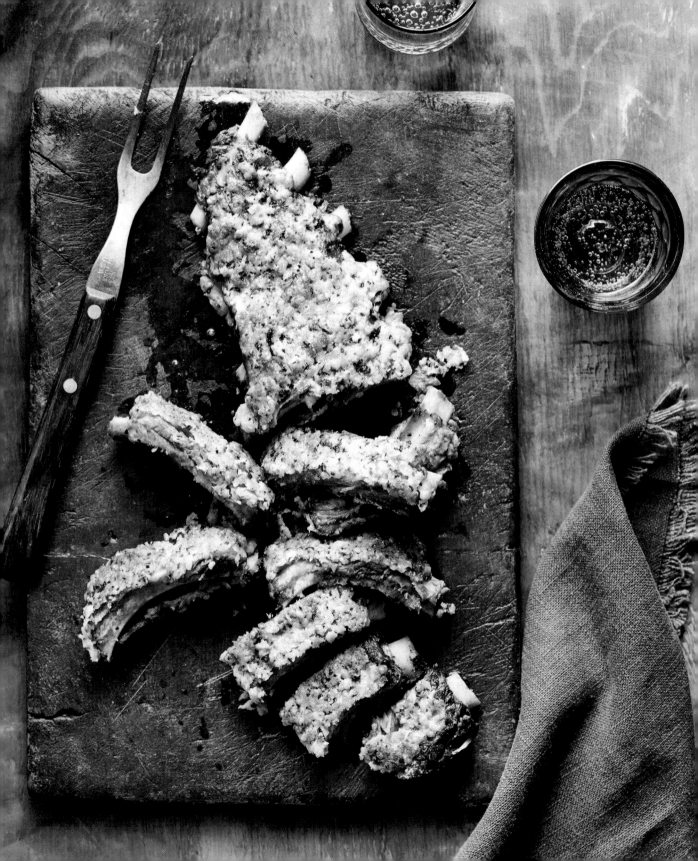

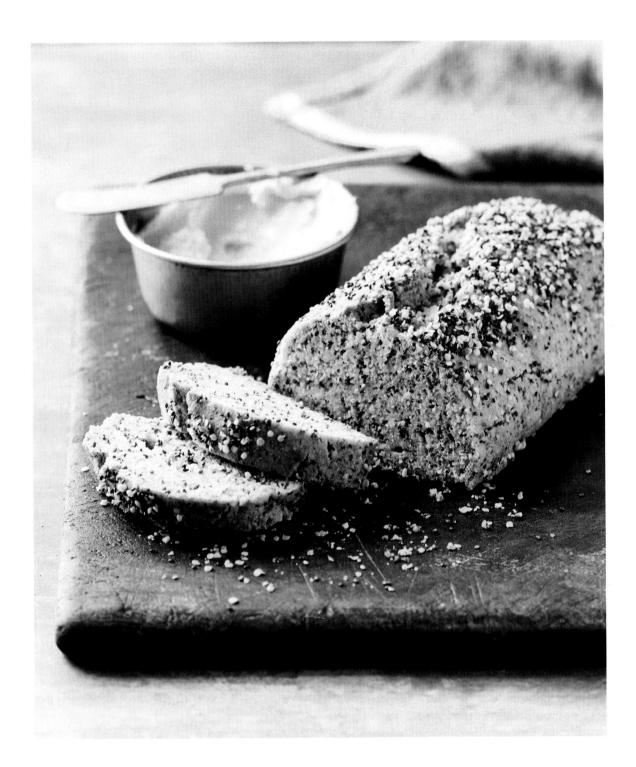

HOMEMADE DRY RANCH SEASONING

¼ cup dried parsley

2 teaspoons garlic powder

2 teaspoons dried dill weed

1 teaspoon pink Himalayan salt

1 teaspoon onion powder

½ teaspoon black pepper

MAKES ABOUT 7 TABLESPOONS

You will use this a lot, so double the recipe and you'll be sure to have some on hand when you need it.

COMBINE all the ingredients in a food processor and pulse until the mixture is combined. Store in a covered container at room temperature for up to 4 months.

NUTRITIONAL INFO (PER 1½ TABLESPOONS)
CALORIES 20, **FAT** 0.2g, **PROTEIN** 1.1g, **CARBS** 4.5g, **FIBER** 1.3g

Note: *To make a smaller batch for just one or two recipes, use the amounts as follows: 1 tablespoon dried parsley, ½ teaspoon garlic powder, ½ teaspoon dried dill weed, ¼ teaspoon pink Himalayan salt, ¼ teaspoon onion powder, and ⅛ teaspoon black pepper. This makes about 1½ tablespoons seasoning.*

HOMEMADE RANCH SALAD DRESSING

½ cup mayonnaise

½ cup sour cream

¼ cup lemon juice

2 tablespoons dried parsley

2 teaspoons onion powder

2 teaspoons dried dill

1 teaspoon garlic powder

1 teaspoon Himalayan pink salt

½ teaspoon black pepper

MAKES 1¾ CUPS (28 SERVINGS)

Loved by both kids and adults, this dressing is great on salads or as a dip for raw vegetables.

COMBINE all the ingredients in a blender and blend on high speed until smooth and creamy. Store in a covered container in the refrigerator for up to 7 days.

NUTRITIONAL INFO (PER 1-TABLESPOON SERVING)
CALORIES 51, **FAT** 4.9g, **PROTEIN** 0.4g, **CARBS** 1.2g, **FIBER** 0.1g

CHAYOTE COMPOTE

3 chayote squash, peeled, seeded, and cut into ½-inch pieces

3 tablespoons Swerve brown sugar sweetener

2 teaspoons lemon juice

1 teaspoon ground cinnamon

½ teaspoon maple extract

½ teaspoon vanilla extract

¼ teaspoon salt

½ teaspoon xanthan gum

MAKES 3 CUPS (6 SERVINGS)

This recipe is amazing poured over your favorite keto ice cream, added to pancakes or waffles, and in the Chayote "Apple" Pie (page 237).

IN a medium pot over medium-high heat, mix together the chayote and 4 cups water and bring to a boil. Lower the heat to medium-low and simmer, adding more water as needed, until the chayote is soft, 35 to 40 minutes. Drain the chayote.

TRANSFER the chayote to a medium skillet over medium heat. Add the sweetener, lemon juice, cinnamon, maple extract, vanilla, salt, and 1 tablespoon water. Cook, stirring frequently, until the sauce has caramelized, about 5 minutes. Sprinkle in the xanthan gum and stir until well combined. Remove from the heat and let cool.

STORE in a covered container in the refrigerator for up to 5 days or freeze for up to 3 months.

NUTRITIONAL INFO (PER ½ CUP)
CALORIES 6, **FAT** 0g, **PROTEIN** 0.2g, **CARBS** 3g, **FIBER** 0.5g

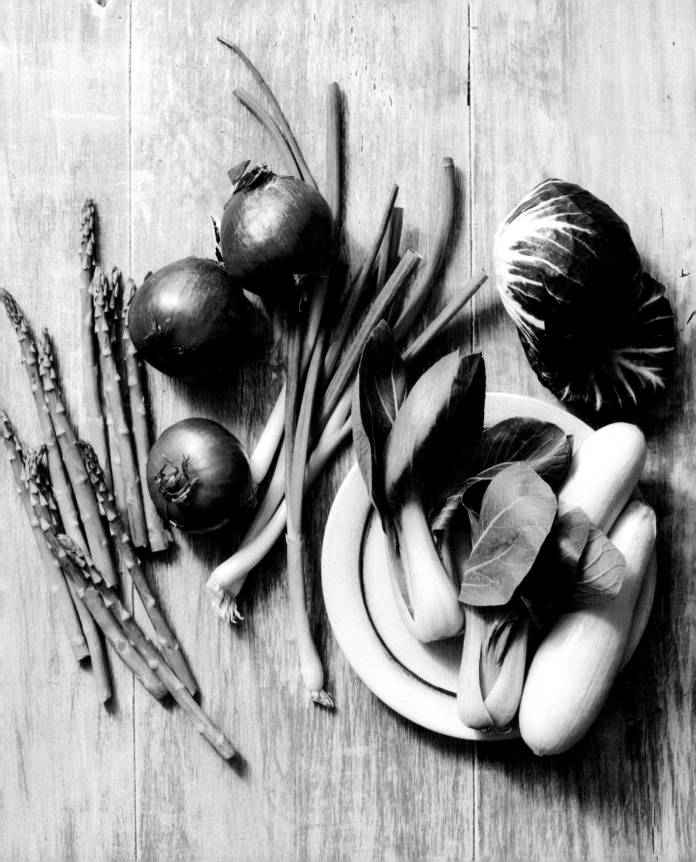

Index

Note: Page references in *italics* indicate photographs.